THE STRUCTURE HOUSE

WEIGHT LOSS PLAN

ACHIEVE YOUR IDEAL WEIGHT THROUGH A NEW RELATIONSHIP WITH FOOD

Gerard J. Musante, Ph.D.

A FIRESIDE BOOK
PUBLISHED BY SIMON & SCHUSTER
New York   London   Toronto   Sydney

This publication contains the opinions and ideas of its author. It is intended to provide help-ful and informative material on the subjects addressed in the publication. It is sold with the understanding that the author and publisher are not engaged in rendering medical, health, or any other kind of personal professional services in the book. The reader should consult his or her medical, health, or other competent professional before adopting any of the sug-gestions in this book or drawing inferences from it.

The author and publisher specifically disclaim all responsibility for any liability, loss or risk, personal or otherwise, which is incurred as a consequence, directly or indirectly, of the use and application of any of the contents of this book.

FIRESIDE
A Division of Simon & Schuster, Inc.
1230 Avenue of the Americas
New York, NY 10020

Copyright © 2007 by Structure House, Inc., and Mel Parker Books LLC

All rights reserved, including the right to reproduce this book or portions thereof in any form whatsoever. For information address Fireside Subsidiary Rights Department, 1230 Avenue of the Americas, New York, NY 10020.

First Fireside trade paperback edition January 2008

FIRESIDE and colophon are registered trademarks of Simon & Schuster, Inc.

Structured Eating is a registered service mark of Structure House, Inc.

For information regarding special discounts for bulk purchases, please contact Simon & Schuster Special Sales at 1-800-456-6798 or business@simonandschuster.com.

Designed by Jan Pisciotta

Manufactured in the United States of America

10   9   8   7   6   5   4   3   2

The Library of Congress has cataloged the hardcover edition as follows:
Musante, Gerard J.
    The structure house weight loss plan : achieve your ideal weight through a new relationship with food / Gerard J. Musante.
        p.   cm.
    Includes bibliographical references and index.
    1. Weight loss.   2. Reducing diets.   3. Nutrition.   I. Title.
RM222.2.M87   2007
613.2'5—dc22   2006051451

ISBN-13: 978-0-7432-8690-9
ISBN-10   0-7432-8690-1
ISBN-13: 978-0-7432-8691-6 (pbk)
ISBN-10   0-7432-8691-X (pbk)

To all the men and women
who have come to Structure House
over the years

Contents

PART III: STAY STRUCTURED:
Maintain the Structure House Weight Loss Plan

Introduction

This is a book about change. I don't mean just change in your weight—losing the pounds you want to lose. Weight loss is important, but it's not really the change that is most important. Rather, *The Structure House Weight Loss Plan* focuses on changing yourself in deeper, more significant, more durable ways than what you can measure simply by standing on your bathroom scale. I'm talking about changing how you view yourself. Changing your relationship with food. Changing your choices about how to live your life. Changing your attitude about change itself.

For thirty years, I've helped overweight and obese men and women learn about change at Structure House, the residential program I founded in Durham, North Carolina. Approximately one thousand people participate in our programs there each year. Some of these participants are ten, twenty, thirty pounds over their desired weight. Others are carrying even more excess pounds and would be considered obese. Still others are morbidly obese—so overweight that their health is in immediate jeopardy. Almost all of the people who come to Structure House understand that excess weight can lead to medical problems such as diabetes, cardiovascular disease, hypertension, and other serious health risks. These participants stay at Structure House for a period of time and, each in his or her own way, learn about the possibilities for change and about the skills that make change possible.

Here are just a few comments from participants about what they gained from the Structure House program:

"Structure House changed my life. It was the best investment I ever made in myself."

—Pete*

"With the information and the tools that I received at Structure House, losing weight is a challenge that I can face. Now I understand my weight problem, and I know what I can do to effectively deal with it."

—Nancy

"To be looked at as a 'normal-weight' person by others instead of always being stared at is a wonderful benefit to my weight loss. I have more energy and I'm in better shape than most of my friends. This lifestyle change has truly given me a new life."

—Jeremy

"Since leaving Structure House I have exercised on a daily basis and generally live a healthy lifestyle. With the training and behavior modification used by Structure House, I am now able to control my food intake and maintain a 'normal' weight."

—Alan

"I have learned how to take better care of myself and am learning how to value myself with a new body and a new approach to food. The program has been, for me, a gift."

—Maria

Structure House is a residential program, but the *concepts* we teach there are flexible, adaptable, and portable. I see Structure House primarily as a *school for change*—a place where participants can stay with us for a while, become Students of Change, acquire as many new skills as possible, then take their skills back home to practice and apply. My purpose in writ-

* All names of participants quoted throughout this book have been changed to protect their privacy.

ing *The Structure House Weight Loss Plan* is to put these concepts into a book so that you can learn and use them in the comfort and familiarity of your own surroundings.

But before we start discussing the Structure House program and its many benefits, I want to touch on some of the issues that inspired me to design this program in the first place.

IT ISN'T *FOOD* THAT MAKES YOU FAT

"I also learned a lot about some of the triggers for *why*
I eat."

—Jack

Each of us has a relationship with food. We all need a certain amount of sustenance to stay alive and healthy, but satisfying our nutritional needs isn't the only reason we eat. From childhood on, every person develops a set of expectations, habits, associations, and states of mind related to food. Our family dynamics, our cultural backgrounds, and our individual attitudes and tastes all influence how this situation develops. We could call the sum total of these expectations, habits, associations, and states of mind our "relationship" with food.

For many people, that relationship is fundamentally healthy. For some, though, the relationship is more complex and even problematic. The kinds and quantities of food we eat may work against our best interests. Some people eat more out of habit than from nutritional need. Some use food as a drug—a substance they take to relax, stimulate, console, or anesthetize themselves. Some view food as a companion that soothes a sense of loneliness or else substitutes for human interaction or other satisfying activities.

One part of the Structure House approach is to help you understand that, like many people, you've learned to use food in ways that go beyond its nutritional value. That's why I say that it isn't *food* that makes you fat. Your problem isn't so much food as such, and it's not even the weight you gain from food; rather, the problem is your *relationship* with food. *Weight is a symptom of an underlying imbalance in your relationship with food.*

When your relationship with food gets out of balance—and when you habitually use food to meet nonnutritional needs—you're going to gain weight. Other negative changes may result from this imbalance, too. Your health may suffer. You may become less physically active. You may start to isolate yourself socially. You may struggle with your sense of self-worth. Sometimes you feel as though you've lost control and there is nothing that you can do to improve your life.

But if you can regain a sense of balance, you'll reap all kinds of benefits. First of all, you'll lose weight—but weight loss is just the start. Your health will begin to improve. You'll lower your risk of cardiovascular disease, diabetes, and joint problems. You'll feel livelier and more active. With more energy available, you'll be more likely to exercise, which will help you lose weight faster and boost your energy and stamina even more. You'll look better, too. And all of these positive changes will bolster your social confidence, your sense of self-worth, and your trust in what life has to offer.

These issues of balance and imbalance have convinced me that real change—not just the change you see on the dial on your bathroom scale—is what matters most. Imbalanced use of food is a behavior you've learned in the past. What you've learned in one way can be unlearned, and you can now learn to have a different, more balanced relationship with food. In short, you can *change*.

I invite you to start this journey—and to experience all the benefits that change can bring you.

PART I

GET STRUCTURED

Understand and Prepare for
the Structure House
Weight Loss Plan

CHAPTER 1

The Structure House Program

We live in an age of reflexive finger-pointing. If you have a problem, someone is to blame. And we're often quick to blame someone *else*. If we're driving somewhere and crash the car, the accident is surely the other driver's fault! (Or the car company's fault—or else the town's fault for not putting up a sign or a traffic light!) To be sure, problems sometimes *do* result from what other people have done or failed to do, but it's also true that people frequently cast blame elsewhere first and only later consider their own possible contribution to the problem.

Unfortunately, this tendency to point fingers—to cast the blame outward rather than look to ourselves for some degree of responsibility—holds true regarding food, weight gain, and weight loss. How many times have you heard people blame external factors for their overweight? Food has too much fat . . . or too many carbs . . . or too many calories. The portions are too large . . . the packages are too big . . . Or else people say they don't have enough time to eat properly . . . or their clothes are just too tight. Or perhaps the problem isn't food, it's exercise—and once again the blame lies elsewhere. There isn't enough time to keep fit . . . Or the ways of staying fit are too difficult . . . too boring . . . too expensive . . . too complicated . . . too *whatever*. Eating too much, not eating right, or not exercising—these can't possibly be factors that *you* have responsibility for, can they? That *you* have some control over?

But there's a major problem with this attitude. If you define a problem as out of your control, you put yourself in a position of being powerless to solve it. This principle is just as true for weight loss as it is for anything else. Is your overweight the result of something Out There? Bad foods? High fat? High carbs? Greedy companies? Purveyors of junk food? Not likely. Almost all experts acknowledge that overweight ultimately results from violating a simple principle: that calories consumed should equal calories expended. If you consume more calories than you expend, you'll gain weight. If you consume fewer calories than you expend, you'll lose weight. It's not something outside you that creates an imbalance in this equation. The idea that the food industry or the toxic environment is victimizing you presents a problem. The reason: this approach stymies your motivation and thus your ability to control your weight.

So if finger-pointing and blame casting don't offer good approaches to weight control, what would be more effective?

My recommendation: Take personal responsibility.

Here's why.

TAKE CONTROL OF YOUR SITUATION

During my several decades of work at Structure House, I've observed that the people who most consistently succeed at losing weight and improving their health are those who take responsibility for their personal situations. They're much more likely to make a serious commitment to change. They're more likely to work hard at reaching their goals. They're also more likely to perceive the connection between their efforts and what they accomplish.

A powerful concept sums up the very human stories I've witnessed over the years at Structure House. A noted Stanford University psychologist, Albert Bandura, defined this concept in 1977 and called it "self-efficacy." Bandura theorized that people's expectations of their ability to be effective determine whether they take action or not. Self-efficacy affects how much effort they expend and how long they will sustain their efforts when confronting challenges. If you feel that the choices you make and the actions you take can influence the outcome of events, you will feel confident in your ability to create change. But if you believe that you're overwhelmed and helpless in the face of external circumstances, you won't feel any confidence in your own capacity to foster change or improve your situation. To put it bluntly: self-efficacy helps you feel in control; lack of self-efficacy leaves you feeling powerless.[1]

For this reason, blaming overweight and obesity on external forces misses the most crucial point. Doing so weakens rather than strengthens your ability to lose weight and improve your health. Blaming factors outside yourself will probably leave you feeling helpless. And if you feel helpless, are you likely to make a commitment to losing weight? I don't think so. Even if you do, you'll tend to ascribe any success you achieve to those powerful outside forces that you feel are in control: special diet foods, proprietary vitamins, "miracle" approaches, and so forth. You won't feel so great *even if you succeed*—because, after all, it's not *your* actions that have led to success!

Instead, take responsibility. This is the first step on your journey toward change. Is responsibility a burden? Not at all! It's the start of a wonderful voyage. You're not a slab of driftwood tossed about on the sea—you're the captain of your fate. If you take control of your situation, you can chart your own course, enjoy the trip, and proudly take credit for success when you reach your destination.

Taking responsibility makes you less vulnerable, not more so. It'll be *you* who's making the choices. If you're the one who's choosing what, when, and why you eat, you're much more likely to have a balanced relationship with food.

Taking responsibility makes you stronger, not weaker. It'll be *you* who's in control. You'll be more likely to make good decisions about meals, exercise, and health care issues.

Taking responsibility gives *you* a clear sense of volition. You'll take control of your situation, and, by doing so, you'll learn, grow, and develop as a person.

THE RISKS OF A FAD-DIET MIND-SET

"In the past [I was] under a doctor's care for weight loss. He prescribed a variety of pills that totally played with my emotions and system. The weight came off—but the moment I stopped taking the pills, the weight went back on again, because I'd never dealt with the underlying issues of why I used food as I did."

—Sallie

You've heard about them. You've probably even tried a few. Fad diets are everywhere—advertised in magazines, discussed on TV, and promoted in books and instructional videos. Scarcely a week goes by without some new diet "guru" claiming that a new method or supplement or weight loss secret will cause your excess pounds to melt away and never come back. There are diets based on catchy concepts: the Eat Great, Lose Weight diet; the Fit for Life diet; the New Beverly Hills Diet; and the Eat Right 4 Your Type diet. There are diets based on eating only one food or just a few: the Grapefruit Diet, the Fruit Juice Diet, and the New Cabbage Soup Diet. There are diets based on liquid meal replacements, such as Slim-Fast and Optifast. There are diets based on dietary supplements—chitosan, senna, chromium picolinate, you name it. There are diets guaranteed to "rid your body of cellulite," to "sweat off the pounds," or to "make the pounds melt away." There are also high-protein, low-carbohydrate diets of all kinds: the Carbohydrate Addicts' Diet, the Zone Diet, the Sugar Busters Diet, the Atkins Diet, the Protein Power Diet, and the South Beach Diet. If these diets aren't extreme enough, some proponents suggest outright fasting—not eating at all. These are all examples of what I call pharmaceutical nutrition: approaches that perceive food as a chemical formulation.

Like many people, you may feel under siege from all sorts of diet advice. Perhaps your relatives call you to suggest a new weight loss pill they've heard about. Your friends pressure you to sample a nutritional supplement that did wonders for them. Your coworkers want you to visit the doctors who helped them lose weight easily. And of course ads on TV, in magazines, and on the Web push all kinds of products, each touted as a miracle cure.

Unfortunately, these fads are all simplistic, and they don't work well over the long term. Why? Because *short-term success may occur as the result of a diet, pill, or surgical procedure, but it won't resolve your long-term problem.* Diets themselves actually have no special power. There's no proof that the specific composition of a diet can lead anyone to success in losing weight and maintaining that loss. By following a fad diet, you probably will lose weight—but you probably won't keep the weight off for long.

There's another issue to consider: fad diets may also damage your confidence in yourself. You may believe that a diet has some sort of special power and that the diet itself will grant the success you crave. When the diet doesn't work out in the long term, though—and they almost always don't—you'll tend to see yourself as the cause of your failure. You may conclude that you can't control the situation and that you can't build the confidence to develop and master the skills that will lead you to success. You'll blame yourself rather than the diet.

Fad diets claim to provide you with the answer (often a simplistic answer), but they don't even ask the right question. These many programs, products, and cures all share a common flaw: they encourage you to expect results based on external cure-alls rather than your own insight and self-mastery. They focus *only* on weight loss. They never address the underlying imbalances that make you vulnerable to using food inappropriately. And until you examine and explore those imbalances, you can't really take steps to reduce your imbalance. You won't be able to acquire the important skills that lead to altering your thoughts, feelings, and behaviors.

WHAT IS THE STRUCTURE HOUSE PROGRAM?

"I like the holistic approach to obesity—addressing not just the physical but the emotional, mental, and spiritual as well. My lifestyle has changed dramatically."

—Janie

At Structure House, we've helped thousands of people become Students of Change and undertake a program that takes the long view, provides a new set of skills, and offers help in using those skills to make long-lasting changes. Unlike what happens when you use the various fad diet approaches, you gain both immediate benefits *and* the ability to accumulate long-term benefits.

The key to the Structure House program is encompassed within Structured Eating, a problem-solving strategy. Structured Eating means eating nutritious food consumed in appropriate portions three times a day—the eating that you need to meet nutritional requirements and maintain the level of weight you desire. Daily calorie consumption is determined on the basis of each individual's sex, height, weight, medical condition, and age. This is all the nutrition your body needs. Any and all other eating is *unstructured eating* and occurs for nonnutritional reasons. Because unstructured eating is certain to exceed your caloric needs, it's also certain to cause weight gain. (An analogy I often use is that of a gas tank: once you fill up your tank, you don't need more fuel.)

In this way, Structured Eating is a system designed to:

- Isolate unhealthy eating habits
- Determine the "eating triggers" that cause unhealthy eating to occur
- Illuminate how you use food in your life
- Shine a spotlight on your relationship with food
- Show you where you need to make changes—not just in the use of food but also in your lifestyle

Structured Eating is also a tool for raising your consciousness and showing you how food functions in your life. Structured Eating prompts you to isolate the other times *when* you eat and to understand *why* you eat. It also prompts you to set specific, targeted behaviors that will help you reach the goals I've listed.

Later chapters in this book will take you step-by-step through the Structure House program, explain how it works, and provide the information you'll need to adapt it to your life. A few reassurances:

- Structured Eating doesn't mean you have to be perfect!
- Although it's not crucial for you to follow your plan 100 percent, it *is* important to have a plan to follow.
- Structured Eating gradually reveals the multiple psychological and environmental aspects of your unhealthy eating and shows you where you need to focus your attention and energy.

Structured Eating offers both an immediate payoff (initial weight loss) and long-term benefits (ongoing weight loss, effective weight maintenance, and improved overall health). This approach is far more productive than the flash-in-the-pan results that so many fad diets create. Using the Structure House approach, you'll be in control of the situation—not controlled by it. You'll gain power by taking responsibility—and then *you* can take credit for your successes.

Four important strategies are part of the Structure House program:

- Take responsibility, take control—and feel better about yourself.
- Change your mind—and change your life.
- Address your medical issues—and rest easy about your health.
- Change how you exercise—and regain your joy in life.

Let's discuss each of these four strategies.

Strategy 1: Take Responsibility, Take Control— and Feel Better About Yourself

> "You have to make yourself accountable—that's the only way to lose the weight and keep it off."
>
> —Sallie

Many overweight people speak as if food is running the show: "Well, the portions were so huge, I just had to eat everything on my plate," or "Once I started, I kept going till the whole quart of ice cream was gone." Wouldn't it be wonderful to break away from this helpless mind-set? Wouldn't it feel great to *eat to live*, not *live to eat*? Wouldn't it feel great to eat only when you're hungry—to enjoy every bite and feel great about the benefits you'll gain rather than feeling bad about the pounds you would have gained if you overate? Wouldn't it feel terrific to exercise, burn off those extra calories, and live a more active life? Taking responsibility and control will boost your motivation and steer you toward success.

Making a commitment to personal responsibility isn't a burden—it's the key to freedom. Take that key, unlock the door, and leave the confining little room of unproductive habits and behaviors that has been trapping you until now. If you take responsibility, you take control. Responsibility will let you change. And change, as I've noted, is the heart of the Structure House program.

Strategy 2: Change Your Mind—and Change Your Life

> "At Structure House, I learned to change my relationship with food for life. I learned that I don't have to overeat, that emotional needs can be met in far more constructive ways."
>
> —Jeannette

Achieving weight loss goals, keeping the weight off, and addressing weight-related health issues are all processes that require you to change *how you think about eating* and the role that food plays in your life. Ask yourself these questions:

- How do I spend my time?
- How do I reward myself?
- How do I set priorities?
- How do I cope with challenges, stress, and anxiety?

The Structure House program will help you answer these questions in dynamic, creative ways. You'll start thinking of yourself as a Student of Change rather than as a passive victim of forces beyond your control. You'll change your thinking processes, emotions, and behaviors as you apply new strategies to your daily life. "Changing your mind" may sound like an abstract intellectual exercise, but it's not. On the contrary, it's wonderfully practical. Just as athletes, performing artists, and many others must master the "inner game" of their sport or art to succeed, changing how you think about food will help you succeed in attaining weight loss, weight maintenance, and a happier life.

Strategy 3: Address Your Medical Issues—
and Rest Easy About Your Health

> "I should let you know that my blood glucose remains well within the normal range; my cholesterol, LDL, HDL, and triglycerides are where they should be; my blood pressure is normal . . . ; and I am down [in weight] about 80 pounds."
>
> —Alyssa

You've seen the headlines about research linking overweight and health problems. You've probably read some of the articles. Overweight and obese people run increased risks for many diseases and health conditions, including hypertension, type 2 diabetes, elevated cholesterol levels, cardiovascular diseases, stroke, gallbladder diseases, osteoarthritis, sleep apnea, and some types of cancer. In fact, an estimated 300,000 deaths per year in the United States alone can be attributed to obesity-related problems.[2]

Is this how you want to live? Are these the risks you want to run? Of course not. And you don't have to. Many medical studies have now documented that even a relatively modest degree of weight loss has significant benefits for overall health.

- Weight loss as minimal as 5 to 15 percent of total body weight in a person who is overweight or obese reduces the risk factors for some diseases, particularly heart disease. Just a ten-pound weight loss can substantially reduce your risk of disease and improve your overall health.

- Losing even 5 to 7 percent of your body weight will also reduce your risk of developing type 2 diabetes by 58 percent.

- Lifestyle changes can prevent or delay the onset of type 2 diabetes among high-risk adults.

- According to the National Institutes of Health, people who lost ten pounds and maintained the weight loss for two years experienced significant reductions in blood pressure, and fewer of them were subsequently diagnosed with high blood pressure than those not losing weight.

By using the Structure House approach, you can improve your health from the outset—and then start to accumulate health benefits that will last a lifetime.[3]

Strategy 4: Change How You Exercise— and Regain Your Joy in Life

"I learned to exercise, which I'd never done before."

—Jack

Exercise is a natural component of healthy weight control and health maintenance. It's not just about sweat and exertion; it's also about recapturing the feelings of lightness, energy, and strength that you may have experienced in the past—feelings that are your birthright. Regardless of your body type or fitness level, you can find wonderful activities to learn and enjoy.

Do you like being outdoors? Start a walking club with your friends. Do circuits at the local park. Go for a hike in the woods.

Maybe you prefer to exercise indoors. Gyms have now spread nationwide—and many are geared toward "regular folks," not just the fit and buff. Many communities schedule fitness classes at the local high school or community college.

Exercise DVDs and personal equipment offer many stay-at-home alternatives. Dyna-Bands and other inexpensive equipment can provide options for resistance and strength training. Or you can just put a CD on your CD player and dance to the music you love.

Yoga, t'ai chi, tae kwan-do, and other martial arts have now gone mainstream. Many YMCAs and JCCs offer classes in these approaches—as well as dance, Jazzercize, swimming, water aerobics, Gyrokinesis, low-impact step aerobics, and kickboxing.

Any of these forms of exercise will help you lose weight and feel better. The key is to get off the sofa and start moving. You'll be amazed by how fast you'll feel better.

THE JOURNEY

"I have taken away enough tools, resources, and 'food for thought' for a lifetime."

—Janie

"I felt like I was going to college. I was getting a college education in proper living—living in a healthy and safe way to make yourself feel the best you can possibly feel."

—Arthur

"If I wanted to be successful on this journey, I would have to open that door and revisit some things in my past."

—Sallie

The Structure House program is best described as a journey. It's a journey that consists both of small, individual steps as well as a larger voyage.

The small steps are specific, focused changes you can take *now* to help you lose weight *now*.

The larger voyage is a process of self-exploration that will help you see yourself in a new light, understand your relationship with food, and make long-term changes that will help you keep the pounds off and improve your health in profound, lasting ways.

Both the small, individual steps and the larger voyage will change your life. More than thirty thousand women and men have become Students of Change while in residence at Structure House; then they've returned to their families to continue their journeys.

You can take this journey, too.

Let me show you how.

CHAPTER 2

Assess Your Health and Medical Issues

"I was borderline diabetic. I had bad HDL, LDL, and triglycerides. And I probably had high blood pressure."

—Arie

"My cholesterol and triglycerides were both elevated, and my blood sugar had gotten into the prediabetes range."

—Jenny

"I could tell that I was starting to develop some health issues. I was still playing some basketball, but every time I played, I'd begin to hurt. My legs and ankles would hurt at night."

—Jack

If you're overweight, you may have developed weight-related medical conditions. It's crucial to assess these problems before starting any weight loss program. First of all, these problems may be significant threats to your well-being. Also, you may have difficulty focusing on a weight loss program if you're preoccupied with your health issues. Weight loss is important, but you need to examine and monitor the bigger picture, too

My recommendation: be your own medical advocate. Take action on your own behalf by following this three-step approach.

STEP 1: GET A COMPLETE PHYSICAL EXAM

You should get a complete physical exam before starting a weight reduction program, whether it's the Structure House approach or any other. This exam is important for these reasons:

- First, to identify any health issues that may be affecting you.
- Second, to identify any health issues that may:
  - Impede a weight loss program
  - Modify the nature of a weight loss program
  - Affect your physiological or psychological responses to a weight loss program
  - Modify the type or level of exercise you can tolerate as part of a weight loss program

If your physical exam shows that you're in good health, you can proceed with the Structure House program full speed ahead.

If your physical exam identifies any health problems, you're certainly better off knowing about them than remaining unaware. Now you can address and solve them. Since your weight-related conditions improve when you lose excess pounds, you may be able to start the Structure House program right away. But get your physician's advice before you start.

Here are the factors that are of greatest concern to people who are overweight.

Prior Health Issues

Tell your primary care physician or internist about any and all prior health issues, as these may affect any weight loss program you undertake. Discussing these issues is especially important if you have a history of heart disease, diabetes, or hypertension.

Cardiovascular Issues

Before starting any weight loss or exercise program, determine your state of cardiovascular health. Do you have any signs and symptoms of heart disease? Do you show indications of hypertension (high blood pressure)? Does your family include blood relatives who have suffered from cardiovascular disease or stroke?

Endocrine Issues

Many people who are overweight or obese have a heightened risk of diabetes. Do you show signs and symptoms of this disorder? Typical signs and symptoms include:

- Excessive production of urine
- Excessive thirst
- Excessive hunger
- Blurred vision
- Drowsiness
- Increased susceptibility to infection

If so, are you under treatment? If you are diabetic but aren't under treatment, what treatment does your physician suggest?

Another issue is thyroid disorders. Do you show signs and symptoms of hypothyroidism? Typical signs and symptoms include:

- Weight gain
- Constipation
- Inability to tolerate cold
- Dry, coarse, sparse hair
- Dry, coarse, scaly, thick skin

If so, ask your physician how he or she intends to treat this disorder.

Exercise-Related Issues

You should also assess any problems that physical activity may aggravate. You may need to exercise in ways that take joint, muscle, or skeletal problems into account. Make sure that your doctor assesses you for these aspects of your health before you start a weight loss program.

History of Eating Disorders, Alcohol Abuse, or Drug Abuse

Do you have a history of anorexia, bulimia, or any other eating disorders? If so, it's important for your primary care physician or internist to know about what happened in the past, as the situation may interact with the sort of weight loss program you undertake. The same is true for any history of alcohol or drug abuse, as these issues may interact with a weight loss program.

Body Mass Index

You should ask your physician to calculate your body mass index (BMI), a tool for indicating adults' weight status. (If you want to do this calculation yourself, see Appendix 1 of this book. Note: The BMI for children and teens is based on gender- and age-specific charts.) For adults over twenty years old, BMI falls into one of these categories:

- Below 18.5: Underweight
- 18.5–24.9: Normal
- 25.0–29.9: Overweight
- 30.0 and above: Obese

Why is BMI important? Weight alone isn't the only factor to consider in determining your level of risk; you also need to take your height into account. As BMI increases, the risk for some diseases (including cardiovascular disease, high blood pressure, osteoarthritis, and some cancers) also increases.

Lab Screening

Part of your physical exam should include a lab screening that includes the following tests:

- Thyroid evaluation
- Serum glucose (blood sugar level—fasting rate should be less than 100 mg/dL)
- Cholesterol levels, including total cholesterol, HDL, LDL, and triglycerides (total cholesterol should be less than 200)
- Complete blood count (CBC), especially for women who are still menstruating (to rule out anemia and obtain a baseline to monitor possible anemia in the future)

Pregnancy

If you're pregnant, a weight loss program would be hazardous to both you and the fetus. It's crucial that your physical exam rule out pregnancy—by means of a pelvic exam, a pregnancy test, or both—before you begin any weight loss program. And if you *are* pregnant, congratulations! We wish you a safe pregnancy, an uneventful delivery, and a healthy child. You can reconsider weight loss after the child's birth.

STEP 2: ASK YOUR DOCTOR THESE IMPORTANT QUESTIONS

Your physical exam is an invaluable opportunity for your primary care physician to assess your health in general. The information you provide, as well as the exam your doctor performs and the lab tests that he or she requests, will help to identify any concerns that need attention. In addition, your physical exam is a great opportunity for you to ask the doctor questions. This is especially important as you get ready to start a weight loss program.

What would be relevant questions to ask? Here are some suggestions.

Am I in good cardiovascular health?

You need to determine, first and foremost, whether you're in good cardiovascular health. If you are, you'll be far more at ease about losing weight and particularly about exercising. If you're not, you need to identify any problems and seek treatment for them.

How detailed should a cardiovascular assessment be? The answer depends on your age, your health history, your current state of health, your risk factors for heart disease, and perhaps other considerations. For some people, the doctor may limit his or her assessment to the physical exam and some lab tests. For others, the doctor may request other diagnostic procedures, such as a stress (treadmill) test. Let's say that you're an overweight 27-year-old who's in good health overall. Your physician would be less likely to order a stress test for you than for a 57-year-old who weighs the same as you but has some health issues or cardiac risk factors. There's no universal set of recommendations.

For everyone, though, relevant questions should focus on:

- Whether you can safely start an exercise program
- What limitations to the level, nature, or pace of an exercise program you should consider
- Whether you are affected by metabolic syndrome (described in the following section)

What is the state of my endocrine health?

Some people who come to Structure House explain their weight gain as a "glandular condition" or a "thyroid condition." Some of these people may, in fact, be clinically hypothyroid (suffering from a low thyroid level). However, there are very few who fit into this category. And most of them have the condition under control through medication. A thyroid condition shouldn't interfere with weight loss. Two issues that are more common among overweight men and women are diabetes and prediabetes.

I'm mentioning this issue because endocrine (glandular) issues are a factor worth investigating. In and of themselves, endocrine issues don't really explain what may be causing most people's overweight; in fact, for the vast majority, endocrine issues are more likely to be the *result* of overeating. In any case, I recommend that you ask your primary care physician or internist about your state of endocrine health. Specifically:

- **Do you show any indications of diabetes?** A blood glucose level of 126 or higher indicates that you are clinically diabetic. If you are aware that you're diabetic, your physical exam is an opportune time to review your current treatment plan. If you haven't been aware that you're diabetic, you should take this opportunity to plan your treatment.

- **Do you show any signs of prediabetes?** According to the American Diabetes Association, the criterion for a precursor condition called prediabetes is a blood glucose level of 100 to 125 mg/dL. (This figure was recently lowered from the previous level of 126 mg/dL.) If your blood glucose level is at or near this figure, you should immediately discuss the situation with your primary care physician. Lifestyle modifications, including a weight loss program and changes in nutrition, can contribute significantly to preventing prediabetes from progressing to frank diabetes.

- **Do you show any signs (such as on lab tests) of a hypothyroid condition?** Your physician should have a thyroid panel (series of tests) done to rule out this condition. In addition, your family history may be relevant to this aspect of your endocrine health.

Postmenopausal women often experience changes in their endocrine system that may lead to a somewhat slower rate of weight loss. If you fall into this age group, don't worry—you can still succeed in losing weight and improving your health.

Do I show signs and symptoms of metabolic syndrome?

Metabolic syndrome is characterized by a group of metabolic risk factors that increase the likelihood of your developing cardiovascular disease, diabetes, or both. The underlying causes of this syndrome are overweight/ obesity, physical inactivity, and genetic factors. People with metabolic syndrome are at increased risk of coronary heart disease, other diseases related to plaque buildup in artery walls (e.g., stroke and peripheral vascular disease), and type 2 diabetes. You could call metabolic syndrome the interface between endocrine issues and cardiac issues. It's not a disease as such, but rather a cluster of "red flags" that may indicate a heightened risk for cardiovascular disease.

According to the American Heart Association, the presence of three or more of these factors identifies the metabolic syndrome:

- Waist circumference 40 inches or greater for men and 35 inches or greater for women
- Fasting blood serum triglyceride level greater than 150 mg/dL
- Blood HDL cholesterol level less than 40 mg/dL for men, less than 50 mg/dL in women
- Blood pressure equal to or greater than 130/85 mm Hg
- Fasting glucose level equal to or greater than 100 mg/dL

Again, these factors don't indicate a disease as such; rather, they suggest that you have a greater risk of developing diabetes or cardiovascular disease. Given the seriousness of these health problems, it's important for you to identify the presence of metabolic syndrome, then modify any of the risk factors you and your physician identify. The safest, most effective, and preferred way to control metabolic syndrome in overweight and obese people is weight loss and increased physical activity. Other steps for managing metabolic syndrome are also important for patients and their doctors. These include:

- Routine monitoring of body weight; waist circumference, the index for central obesity; blood glucose; HDL and triglyceride levels; and blood pressure
- Treatment of individual risk factors (blood lipids, hypertension, and high blood glucose) according to established guidelines
- Careful choice of antihypertensive drugs, since different medications have different actions within your body to control blood pressure

Are any of my current medications likely to affect my ability
to lose weight safely? And will these medications
affect my ability to exercise safely?

Certain medications may affect a weight loss program, the rate at which you lose weight, and your ability to exercise. You should discuss any medications you are taking with your primary care physician and ask how they may affect you. Here's a partial list of medications that can affect weight loss.

- **Certain cardiovascular medicines.** An example of these: beta-blockers, such as atenolol, Toprol, and Inderal. These medications slow pulse rates and can affect the intensity of exercise.

- **Certain medications for treating diabetes.** Some antidiabetes drugs may actually cause weight gain.

- **Some antidepressants.** These medicines have a common side effect of causing weight gain. Similarly, tricyclic antidepressants, once used to combat depression but now much more likely to be used to treat neuropathies, such as peripheral neuropathy, may also cause you to gain weight.

- **Steroids.** These often contribute to weight gain. Some of this side effect is water retention, but steroids may also stimulate your adrenal glands, thus leading to weight gain.

Taking any of these medications does not mean that you shouldn't go ahead with a weight loss program. But you should discuss the issues with your physician and rely on his or her advice before you make a decision to go ahead.

What is the state of my joints?

When starting a weight loss program, many people overlook the health of their joints. If your joints aren't in good shape, exercise may damage them further. Good overall flexibility, too, is important as you start your weight reduction program.

How do you know if your joints are at risk? It's not just a question of your overall weight. We've had participants at Structure House who weigh 400 pounds or more but have good mobility. Other people weighing less may have far more difficulty. There are many factors that contribute to an individual's joint health, activity level, and mobility. Ultimately, determining a safe level of exercise—and which activities are advisable—should be a result of careful consultation with your primary care physician and, if necessary, with a rheumatologist (joint specialist) as well.

Here are some specific issues to consider:

- **Overall flexibility.** How flexible are your joints, and will your flexibility be adequate for the exercise program you've selected?

- **Knee and hip problems.** Have you suffered damage to your knees and hips, as a consequence of either overweight or other issues?

- **Lower back problems.** Has overweight stressed your lumbar spine or lower back muscles?

- **Arthritis.** Do you have a history of arthritis, and, if so, will it limit the type and amount of exercise you can do?

- **Side effects of injuries** (car accidents, other accidents, or weight-related joint problems). Have you suffered injuries of any sort? To what degree will the side effects of these injuries affect your ability to exercise?

- **Plantar fasciitis.** Do you have a history of this inflammation of tendons in the soles of the feet?

Do I have any other health conditions that might affect me during a weight loss program?

The health issues I've described above are the most common problems that affect people during a weight loss program. However, a few other conditions can also contribute to difficulty losing weight. One to keep in mind is **Stein-Leventhal syndrome or polycystic ovary syndrome (PCOS).** This disorder affects an estimated 6 to 10 percent of all women, most of whom don't know they have it. PCOS is treatable but not curable by means of medication, changes in diet, and exercise. In addition to being one of the leading causes of infertility in women, PCOS can produce the following symptoms:

- Irregular or absent menses (periods)
- Cysts on the ovaries

- High blood pressure
- Weight problems or obesity centered around the midsection
- Elevated insulin levels, insulin resistance, or diabetes
- Excess hair on the face and body
- Thinning of the scalp hair (alopecia)
- Acne

From a standpoint of weight reduction and maintenance, PCOS is most significant because of the issues of high blood pressure, weight around the midsection, and diabetes.

STEP 3: READY, SET, GO

It's easy to postpone facing weight and health problems. Many people do. Millions of Americans deny their own weight issues, ignore them, or choose to eat in ways that make their problems worse. This approach to overweight and weight-related health problems has a name we all know: wishful thinking.

You don't need to live like that. You don't *want* to live like that. Rather than just crossing your fingers, you're better off examining the quality of your life and making some changes.

Rather than ignore reality, I urge you to do what thousands of Structure House participants have done:

- Accept the fact that you have weight issues—and perhaps weight-related medical problems—that need your attention.
- Get a thorough physical exam that identifies any areas of concern—diabetes, cardiovascular problems, and so forth.
- With your physician's guidance, plan a strategy for coping with these problems.
- Based on your primary care physician's or internist's advice, decide whether you should start a weight loss program—including what kind of exercise program you can safely undertake and how strenuous the level of exercise can be.

Once you get the go-ahead, you're ready to Get Structured and take control of your life and your weight.

CHAPTER 3

Get Ready for Structure

"I'd try different diets, but they weren't giving me the tools that I needed. I was busy being perfect on the diet, but I didn't really have any tools to stay there or to address the issues of why I'd eat so much."

—Lisa

"I tried the NutriSystem program. I tried the Cambridge Diet. I was on Weight Watchers and was successful as long as I followed the program. These programs all dealt with food; they didn't deal with emotional issues. The weight came off—but the weight went back on again because I'd never dealt with the underlying issues of why I used food as I did."

—Sallie

"I use food, I guess, to compensate for unhappiness. Well, it gets deeper, because not only was I heavy, I had a marriage that fell apart. My job changed and took a swing to a different direction, and I guess I found food as an escape."

—Aaron

I've heard comments like these from thousands of men and women at Structure House. What they have in common is a poignant truth: you can lose weight on any diet, but it's far harder to keep the weight off. And it's even more unusual for dieters to understand why they eat too much in the first place.

The solution to overweight is Structured Eating, a strategy that helps you meet your nutritional needs without resorting to the problematic, nonnutritional kinds of eating, such as eating out of habit, eating to relieve boredom, and eating to ease stress. Chapters 4 to 6 of this book will explore this strategy and help you Get Structured.

Before we explore the specifics of Structured Eating, however, I recommend that you take six steps that will help you get ready for Structure.

STEP 1: FACE THE PROBLEM

All of us have certain attitudes and opinions. There's no way around this fact—it's just part of human nature. Among other things, we have attitudes and opinions about issues of health, nutrition, weight, and overweight. What we believe is partly the result of diets we may have been on, books we've read, and statements we've heard through the media. Understandably, all this input prompts us to form certain attitudes and opinions.

What I've seen over the years is that the attitudes and opinions people have about health, nutrition, and weight are often incorrect. Maybe you've heard misleading or incomplete information, so you've formed opinions that aren't grounded in facts ("Cabbage contains an enzyme that helps melt away fat"). Maybe your attitudes are so negative that your mind-set will guarantee failure even before you start dealing with your weight issues ("I've never been successful at losing weight before, so why should this time be any different?"). Maybe your opinions and attitudes prevent you from facing the problem in the first place ("I'm not *really* overweight—my clothes are just a bit too tight, that's all").

So the first step in getting ready for Structure is taking a close look and being honest with yourself about your attitudes and opinions about your weight.

Here are some attitudes and opinions that I frequently hear regarding weight and weight loss:

- "I probably have glandular problems, so there's really no point in my changing what I eat, or how often."
- "If I eat only low-fat snacks, there's no way I'll gain any weight."
- "Special combinations of foods will make weight loss easy."
- "Weight loss surgery will solve all my weight problems for good."
- "Since everyone in my family is overweight, there's obviously nothing I can do about my own weight issues."
- "If I take chitosan [or hoodia, or senna, or chromium picolinate], I can eat whatever and whenever I want and know I'll still lose weight."

If you have gathered opinions and attitudes over the years that are incorrect, how should you change them? And by changing them, can you face the problem before you?

The best way to proceed is to ask and answer three important questions.

Question 1: Why do I weigh too much?

In my work at Structure House, I find that most of our participants say outright, "I weigh too much." Saying these words is a necessary first step to facing the problem. However, I've also found that many people hesitate to answer the question *"Why* do I weigh too much?" with full open-mindedness. Suppose I offer two alternative explanations:

1. You weigh too much because your metabolism is unbalanced, or
2. You weigh too much because you eat too much.

Many people will select answer 1.

Which do *you* select?

If you selected 1, you're still not facing the problem. The truth is, *metabolism does not prevent you from losing weight*. Studies haven't proved that becoming overweight is a result of metabolism rather than caloric intake. As I mentioned in Chapter 2, I strongly urge you to undergo a total physical examination, complete with appropriate blood and metabolic tests, to determine that no physical basis exists for your difficulty in controlling your weight. But even if you do have a metabolic condition (such as hypothyroidism), you must still eat less and exercise more in order to lose weight. You can't make the changes necessary for successful weight loss if you believe that metabolic or endocrine problems alone prevent you from losing weight. You must accept that your weight is *in your control* and not *out of your control*.

So when you ask the question "Why do I weigh too much?" the answer—to put it bluntly—is: "I weigh too much because I eat too much."

Question 2: Why do I eat too much?

This question has almost as many answers as there are people who ask it. As I mentioned earlier, each of us has a relationship with food. If you're eating for reasons other than a need for physiological nutrition, the reasons will be highly individual. Here are some of the most common explanations I've heard from Structure House participants over the years:

- "When I get home from work, eating a big snack is how I unwind."
- "Sometimes there's nothing else to do, so I guess eating is basically a form of entertainment."
- "I'm the cook in our family. I'm always nibbling here and there while I'm in the kitchen; all that food is right in front of me!"
- "I like to have some chips while I watch TV. Once I get started, it's hard to stop. Pretty soon the whole bag is gone."
- "If I'm feeling low, food is an emotional boost."
- "At restaurants there are just so many options—and the portions are huge! It's easy to order too much and eat too much."
- "I guess I've always tended to overeat, so now it's hard to stop."

I could quote many others. What's interesting and helpful, though, is seeing that these explanations and all others fall into just three basic categories for nonnutritive eating: habit, boredom, and stress. That's it. If you're overeating, it's for one or another of these reasons. (I'll have lots more to say about this topic in the chapters that follow.)

Question 3: Why didn't my past diets work?

Because your relationship with food is so deeply intertwined with your life and so powerful, *diets alone won't solve your weight problems*. This is true for *everyone*.

Time after time I've heard this question: "Why didn't my past diets work?" Newly arrived participants in our programs tell me, "You name it, I've done it from A to Z. I've tried everything—and I haven't been successful." And because their efforts haven't worked, many people blame themselves for an inability to lose weight or maintain their weight loss.

This kind of self-blame is unfortunate. First of all, feelings of guilt and self-blame really have no place in successful weight control. They don't tell you what to do, what direction to take, where the problem came from, or what's fueling the problem. Guilt and self-blame simply make you feel bad about yourself. I think we can all agree that this approach serves no purpose.

In addition, self-blame doesn't identify *where the problem lies*. Rather than finding fault with yourself, you should try to understand why your previous efforts didn't work. It's not because something was wrong with *you;* instead, something was wrong with the *diets*. The diet approaches were incorrect or incomplete.

Exercise 1: Diet History

Here's how to explore this issue. Take a sheet of paper. Draw a line down the center from top to bottom to create two columns. At the top of the left-hand column, write "All the Diets I've Tried." At the top of the right-hand column, write, "Reasons These Diets Didn't Work." List your past diets in the first column; in the second column, note the reasons they didn't work. (If you need additional space, use more than one page.)

Be honest! Be blunt! If you can face what happened in the past, you can free yourself and move forward to a better, happier future.

All the Diets I've Tried	Reasons These Diets Didn't Work

Now look at the two columns. What's the pattern you see?

Here are three situations typical of what I've read among comments by thousands of Structure House participants in the past.

All the Diets I've Tried	Reasons These Diets Didn't Work
Cabbage Soup Diet	Went on diet, lost 18 lbs., regained all the weight once eating normal food again.
Optifast	Lost weight but didn't like being restricted to all-artificial products. Started regaining weight right after ending diet.
Metabolism Diet	Hated the rigidity of day-to-day plan. Sneaked snacks on the side during diet. Gained weight again after going back on regular diet.

You deserve better outcomes than these! But rest assured: there's nothing wrong with *you*! These diets, not you, are at fault. You haven't been able to control your weight because the previous treatments and diets you have tried have been inadequate. One of the real reasons why diets fail is what I call "diet magic."

The Hazards of "Diet Magic"

Diet Magic occurs when someone—a diet author, a diet guru, whoever—presents you with a formula of foods and claims that this formula will solve all your weight problems. Either directly or by implication, these people tell you, "This is a very special formula. If you eat this combination of foods [or this special food, powder, or liquid], you'll burn fat and lose weight." Here's the truth: researchers in the nutrition field have looked for such a thing as a magic formula in foods for decades now but to no avail. Nobody has found the magic formula. It just doesn't exist.

In addition, there's a common denominator to all of these approaches. It's an obsession: *weight loss as symbolized by the scale.* You're supposed to get on your scale every day. You have a target weight to aim for. Eventually, that scale will show you that perfect number, and when you reach it, your problem will be solved.

Wouldn't it be wonderful if things worked out that way? If you only had to lose weight to solve this problem! But losing weight isn't the whole story. Yes, it's important to lose weight. You want to lose weight. And you *will* lose weight. But the real issue isn't just losing weight—it's *keeping that weight off.* The true issue is lifelong weight management.

Why is ongoing weight management so important? Here's why: *The method you use to lose weight should resemble the method you'll use to manage your weight.* The more similar those two methods are, the greater the likelihood that you'll actually achieve the change you seek. If your *method of weight loss* and your *method of weight management* are pretty much alike, you have a good chance of success. If, on the other hand, your *method of weight loss* and your *method of weight management* are vastly different, your chance of making the leap from one to the other is pretty slim. It's a huge leap to go from eating only a special liquid to eating a regular diet. It's also a huge leap to go from consuming fruit juice, special soups, or any of the many other weight loss gimmicks to eating normal food. These drastic switches are unlikely to succeed. By contrast, the Structure House approach emphasizes weight management from the start so that when the time comes, you'll be well prepared for the transition to maintaining your optimal weight.

STEP 2: UNDERSTAND THAT YOU HAVE A RELATIONSHIP WITH FOOD—AND DISCOVER YOUR "PSYCHOLOGICAL FOOD DNA"

All the miracle pills and perfect food formulas in the world won't solve your weight problems if you don't clarify *why* you eat as well as *what* you eat. But once you understand the reason why, you're on your way to success in weight loss and weight management.

For all of us, food serves nutritional purposes: we eat because our bodies need the nutritional components (protein, carbohydrates, fats, vitamins, minerals, and water) that food provides. But it's also possible to develop a relationship with food that goes beyond nutrition. For instance, most of us experience food partly in social terms. Food is part of family life. Food is also part of our interaction with friends, acquaintances, and coworkers. These are generally normal parts of a person's relationship with food.

Sometimes, however, a relationship with food becomes distorted. It can even get out of control. Sallie, a Structure House participant, describes her relationship with food in these words: "Food has always been my friend, my companion, my lover. It's nonjudgmental. It's always there. I can count on it at any time. And in the past, instead of dealing with the reasons why I was upset or frustrated or unhappy, I turned to food."

Is this statement extreme? It's certainly blunt-spoken and poignant, but over the years I've heard many Structure House participants describe troubled (and troubling) relationships with food, relationships in which food has become the primary source of stimulation: a replacement for friendship, a substitute for love, or a drug that relieves stress, boredom, anxiety, or depression. These sorts of relationships with food make weight loss and weight management a complex task that no quick-fix formula will ever cure.

Here's the truth: Quick-fix diets ignore your relationship with food. If you try to lose weight by popping pills or drinking a special beverage, you're still no closer to understanding why you eat too much under normal circumstances. If you try to lose weight by eating only specific foods, you face the same limits on your insights about why you eat too much. The same holds true if you undergo surgery. Yes, you'll lose weight; as I mentioned earlier, almost all diets produce an initial phase of weight loss. But will you *maintain* the weight loss? Probably not. Most people regain the pounds they've lost. I've seen that disappointing outcome time after time.

That's why the Structure House approach makes the issue of a person's relationship with food central. Here's a brief exercise that will help you see what I'm talking about.

Exercise 2: Is Your Relationship with Food Dysfunctional?[1]

To explore your relationship with food, answer the following questions about how, when, and why you eat. Use the numbers 0 through 4 to indicate your response.

0: No, never
1: No, not very often
2: Occasionally
3: Yes, sometimes
4: Yes, frequently

_____ I eat when I am anxious (nervous).
_____ I cannot control my eating on the weekends.
_____ I eat when people encourage or pressure me to eat.
_____ I eat when I feel physically run down.
_____ I eat when I watch TV.
_____ I eat when I am depressed (or "down").
_____ I eat when there are many different kinds of foods available.

_____ I eat when I feel it would be impolite to refuse a second helping.

_____ I eat when I have a headache.

_____ I eat when I am reading.

_____ I eat when I am angry or irritable.

_____ I eat when I am at a party.

_____ I eat when other people pressure me to eat.

_____ I eat when I am in pain.

_____ I eat just before going to bed.

_____ I eat when I experience failure.

_____ I eat when high-calorie foods are available.

_____ I eat when I think other people will be upset if I don't eat.

_____ I eat when I feel uncomfortable.

_____ I eat when I am unhappy.

Now let's score your answers. There's no "correct" score as such; rather, this exercise serves to suggest the nature of your relationship with food. Note the number of times you wrote 3 and 4 as you answered the questions. The more 3s and 4s you put down, the more often you're using food for nonnutritive reasons. A high frequency of 3s and 4s indicates a relationship with food in which food serves these purposes:

- Easing stress and anxiety
- Relieving sadness and depression
- Providing a substitute for relationships with other people
- Filling the gaps in activities and pastimes
- Providing an outlet for anger and frustration
- Easing tension
- Taking up time when nothing else is happening
- Easing social anxieties
- Offering consolation for rejection
- Soothing physical or emotional pain
- Providing entertainment
- Distracting you from unpleasant, confusing, or threatening emotions

I need to emphasize strongly that if your relationship with food includes these nonnutritive kinds of eating, it doesn't mean that you've done something bad or wrong. Unfortunately, it's common for overweight men and women to be judgmental about themselves—to feel guilty and ashamed about their patterns of eating. That's understandable; it's what our culture has pressed upon us. I hope you can set aside these emotions and attitudes! *Nothing I'm telling you now has to do with being "good" or "bad."* It's certainly understandable that you or anyone else might use food to ease stress, relieve sadness, fill the gaps in your activities, and so forth. Food is cheap and readily available. It is enjoyable. It *does* offer a means of addressing the often difficult situations I've noted. So it's not at all surprising that millions of people use food for nonnutritive purposes. What we're discussing, though, is how food can take a disproportionate place in your life. Food certainly can serve purposes beyond simply fueling your body. Your parents' approaches to food during your childhood (meals, snacks, "rewards") as well as cultural customs (traditional foods, holiday goodies), can all affect your relationship with food. These are understandable "contributions" to your relationship with food. But when your relationship with food becomes excessive—and when you resort to nonnutritive eating often and over a long period of time, what started out as a solution to a problem (stress, sadness, boredom, and so forth) can become a problem in its own right (overweight and health issues). It's those problems that require our attention.

Now let's take your exploration a step further. Why do you have this relationship with food? Why has food become so important that it affects your life in negative ways?

To answer these questions, think about these aspects of how food fits into your personal, family, and community settings:

- **From birth onward, food "feeds" you in more ways than what's obvious.** During your infancy, for instance, your mother may have breast-fed you—an experience that was part of your first and most basic bond with another human being. During babyhood, toddlerhood, and childhood, food was also a fundamental and crucial part of your life. Food remains part of your experience of belonging later in life, too. (I'll bet you don't refer to certain favorite meals as "comfort food" just because they meet your nutritional requirements!)

- **Food is "bait"—and a Band-Aid.** How often during your childhood did your mother and father coax, cajole, threaten, console, or tempt you with food? Use of food for these purposes is common, and it often creates patterns of nonnutritive eating. Here are just a few examples:

- "I know you're upset. Let's have some ice cream so you'll feel better."
- "If you don't eat your vegetables, you can't have dessert."
- "You've been so naughty I won't let you eat your candy."
- "Finish your dinner like a good girl."
- "Stop crying and I'll give you a cookie."

The reward/punishment uses of food can establish patterns of how food affects you emotionally through childhood and into adulthood.

- **Food is one of the "ties that bind."** Adolescence and adulthood also include many experiences in which food has a central place well beyond the family. Work and social settings alike frequently emphasize the importance of food. When you were a teenager, was food part of your social life with peers? Of course. In college, did food fit into campus life—study sessions, dorm parties, and sports events? Of course. Now that you're an adult, what would a staff party at work be like without food? Just imagine.

- **Food is an ongoing focal point of family life.** Although fewer families eat meals together on a regular basis than in the past, the family dinner table remains an American icon. Sharing meals remains an ideal that people aspire to and acknowledge as important even when they can't attain it.

- **Rituals and celebrations include "breaking bread together."** No matter what your ethnic or religious background, you probably put food front and center at holiday times. Thanksgiving, Christmas, Hanukkah, Easter, Passover, Kwanzaa, and Eid al-Fitr (the end of Ramadan) are all big food fests. The same is true with most rites of passage: Bar and Bat Mitzvahs, First Communion celebrations, and other religious occasions all highlight food as part of the occasion. So do weddings and birthday parties.

- **Many activities include food as an enjoyable component.** Think of what sports events would be like without food. ("Buy me some peanuts and crackerjack, / I don't care if I never come back.") Even if you just stay home and watch games on TV, you probably have some munchies close at hand. The same holds true at other kinds of home get-togethers—card games, book clubs, and watching DVDs.

I think you'd agree that all of these experiences can have a major impact on your life. It's no wonder that each of us has a relationship with food that goes beyond nutrition alone. I call the long-term influences of this situation *psychological food DNA*. By this I mean the cumulative, deep impact that food has on our personalities—the sum total of our experiences with food. Here are some examples.

- Throughout Jane's childhood, her mother routinely used food as a source of solace, distraction, and comfort whenever her daughter faced a problem of any sort. Candy was part of the "treatment" for a skinned knee or any other minor injury. An ice cream cone was the consolation for losing the school spelling bee. Extra helpings at dinner served to compensate for a low mood. As a result of numerous experiences, Jane learned to see food as the "cure-all" for her life's discomforts, hurts, and setbacks. Now, during adulthood, she still responds to personal crises—at work, in her marriage, in her role as a mother, and elsewhere—by "medicating" herself with food.

- Stuart didn't have early experiences like Jane's, but his family influenced him in other ways. Raised in the rural Northwest, his parents struggled financially for many years. Food wasn't always abundant—or even sufficient. Stuart grew up with a fear of never having enough to eat. Now prosperous and middle-aged, he is in no danger of malnourishment. Because he equates abundant food with security, however, his early experiences often prompt him to overeat.

- Mariella grew up in a large family whose cultural background puts a high premium on hospitality and abundance at every meal. Her parents considered it important to "put out a big spread," especially at dinnertime, and it was equally important for members of the family to "eat hearty." Her background has strongly affected Mariella's tendency to equate eating (and overeating) with emotional well-being.

As a result of situations like these, you can see how your psychological food DNA is the deeply established pattern of how you respond to food as a result of your personal past.

The impact of what I'm describing is understandable. The situation is by no means all negative. As Thanksgiving, other holidays, and any number of ordinary family and community occasions demonstrate, food is a central and often wonderful part of our lives. It's *good* to enjoy food and the personal, family, and cultural pleasures that it allows us. But some factors can combine to complicate this generally positive situation and make it burdensome in the long run. If your relationship with food emphasizes *a reliance on nonnutritive eating*, it may become a dysfunctional behavior rather than a creative force in your life. Your relationship with food may be intangible and subtle—something, in fact, that you're not even fully aware of—but it can still undermine your state of health and your state of mind. For some people, the damage is physical: overweight and the weight-related risks of high blood pressure, elevated cholesterol, or diabetes. For others, the impact is emotional rather than physical: low self-esteem, depression, anxiety, guilt, severe shyness, or even social phobia. For still others, the impact is both physical and emotional.

But you're now concerned enough about these risks that you've bought this book. You've decided to face the problem. Congratulations on your honesty and courage! By understanding your relationship with food—where it came from, why it exists, and what's maintaining it—you'll greatly increase your ability to lose weight and maintain your weight loss.

Here's another factor that's important: there are as many different relationships with food as there are individual human beings. No two of these relationships are alike. Just as all the other relationships in your own life are unique—your relationships with your parents, your siblings, your children, your other relatives, your coworkers, your neighbors, and your friends—your relationship with food, too, is unique. Why is this uniqueness important? Because it means that you can't just take a method "off the shelf" and assume that it's going to have the same benefits for you as it had for someone else. You can't say, "Well, the [fill in the blank] diet worked for them, so I'm sure it'll work for me." Now that you've made a commitment to change, you can undertake an individual search and see what works for *you*. Take control of the situation! Shift from a dysfunctional relationship with food to a healthy one.

STEP 3: GET READY TO LEARN—
AND UNLEARN

Your relationship with food is something you've *learned*. Is this a cause for alarm? Not at all! Viewing your relationship with food as learned behavior provides a hopeful, powerful way of looking at the situation. If you've learned a certain pattern of behavior, you can also unlearn it. You can learn new ways—better ways—of coping with food. You can take control of this aspect of your life.

Here are two examples—one individual, the other more general— about learning and unlearning.

Ned and Jessie, a couple in their early forties, have both struggled with weight issues for many years. There are many reasons for their having a weight problem, but one of them is their use of food to relieve stress. When they're feeling pressured or anxious, both Ned and Jessie resort to snacking as a "safety valve." Ned prefers salty snacks, such as chips and pretzels. Jessie tends to eat ice cream when under stress. Husband and wife "aid and abet" each other in snacking—either by ignoring the other's habit or even by contributing to the situation through joint sessions of nibbling. As a result, both have gained weight, partly because of this aspect of their relationship with food. But they recently came up with an alternate method of relieving stress: they give each other back rubs. This arrangement isn't always feasible (such as when one member of the couple is at work), but it's effective at home and often helps to ease their craving for food. I think you'd agree that back rubs have a much lower caloric value than a pint of Chunky Monkey or a bag of Doritos. What Ned and Jessie have done changes only one aspect of their relationship with food, but it's definitely a good change, and it serves this couple well.

The second example is culturewide rather than just individual. I believe that our food preferences are often learned. Just four or five decades ago, two specific foods I'm thinking about were far outside of mainstream American culture. In fact, these two foods showed up almost exclusively in ethnic neighborhoods, often in our country's larger cities. Most Americans didn't have a taste for these foods. Which two foods am I referring to? One of them is pizza; the other is bagels. No longer confined to Italian or

Jewish neighborhoods, these foods are now available throughout the United States. You can find them in any supermarket anywhere in this country. Our culture has adopted these foods and made them part of mainstream culture. As a result, people who previously would never have considered eating a bagel or a slice of pizza—and who might never even have heard of them—have now learned to adapt these foods to their own menus and often feel a craving for them.

Look into your heart and ask yourself two questions: "Do I have certain food likes and dislikes?" and "Are some of these likes and dislikes detrimental to my long-term success?" I think you'll admit that you *do* have preferences—and that some of these preferences have negative consequences. If you answer, "Well, I don't like fruits and vegetables, but I sure like candy, cake, and ice cream," I'm sure you'll agree with me that you'll have an uphill battle as you deal with weight and weight-related problems. But you can stare down the reality of these preferences and deal with them. You *can* do that; you *can* relearn your responses to specific foods—and change your overall relationship with food.

STEP 4: UNDERSTAND WHY THIS PROBLEM IS SO COMPLEX

Over the past thirty years, participants have come to Structure House from all fifty states in America and thirty-six other countries. These people are intelligent, talented, and capable. Yet time and time again I've heard folks say, "You know, I just don't understand this. I've been successful at everything else I've done except for solving this one problem! But this one defeats me. Why is that?" Well, it's a good question—one that's important to ask and answer. Unless you can come to understand how complex this problem is—how multilayered it is—you're much less likely to succeed at the tasks you need to undertake.

You Don't Become Overweight Overnight!

By reading this book, you're making a statement: "I weigh too much." But I don't believe that you discovered your weight problem just this past Sunday morning. I don't believe that you got up, looked in the mirror, and exclaimed, "Oh, my God, I'm overweight! What happened to me? Maybe it was something I ate last night!" Weight problems don't happen overnight; they accumulate over an extended period of time. You've eaten too much over time, so now you weigh too much. That's a connection you need to make. For all the talk about metabolism and genetics, the truth is that you've taken in more calories than your body requires to maintain a desired weight.

But here's the key: No form of human behavior occurs in a vacuum. Let me say that again: *No form of human behavior occurs in a vacuum.* When you overeat and gain too much weight, other events begin to occur in the overall context of your life. One of the events that occurs is that you may stop doing certain things that used to be habitual. Even if you gain just ten or fifteen pounds, exercising may appeal to you less than before. This happens for two reasons. One is that as you gain weight, certain actions that you used to perform easily may become more difficult—actions like climbing a flight of stairs or going for a walk. In addition to these physical changes, you may experience psychological changes: you may stop *wanting* to do things. You don't *want* to climb the stairs. You don't *want* to go for a walk. You may pull back from social engagements because you feel more self-conscious about your appearance.

These changes are often gradual. They aren't necessarily major changes at first. But if you don't deal with overeating, and if you stop exercising, the changes often accelerate and accumulate. You're gaining weight—and you wonder if other people can see that you're gaining weight, too. You're uneasy because you suspect that people sometimes stare at you. You worry that your clothes don't seem to fit right. You don't like to look at yourself in the mirror anymore. You wonder if anyone notices how much you sweat when everyone else seems comfortable. And how does that uncertainty make you feel? Not so great. Worst of all are how changes to your body affect your sense of self. Just as visible results are accumulating, some invisible results are accumulating, too. These are "invisible" results in the sense that you know they're there, but no one else does. If you are overeating and gaining weight, invisible results probably include negative thoughts: "Something must be wrong with me," "I lack character," "I lack backbone," "I'm so terrible." These are all statements that

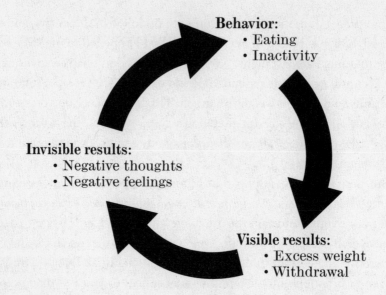

Behavior:
- Eating
- Inactivity

Invisible results:
- Negative thoughts
- Negative feelings

Visible results:
- Excess weight
- Withdrawal

I've heard people make about themselves over the years. So many negative feelings! And, of course, if you're experiencing such intense discomfort, you're probably craving relief. And how do you spell relief? F-O-O-D!

The above diagram shows you the sequence I'm describing:

- **Behavior** (such as *overeating* and *inactivity*) leads to . . .
- **Visible results** (such as *excess weight* and *withdrawal*), which lead to . . .
- **Invisible results** (such as *negative thoughts* and *negative feelings*), which lead to . . .
- **Behavior** (*overeating* and *inactivity*), which leads to . . .

Before you know it, you find yourself caught up in the vicious cycle. For many people, this vicious cycle gains momentum and energy over time, just like a hurricane! That's why sometimes people describe this situation as a "whirlpool" that draws them under. It's a powerful problem. You have the power within you to break this cycle. With the program that I will outline for you in this book, you can change your relationship with food, lose your excess weight, and understand the keys to managing and maintaining your weight.

STEP 5: ACCEPT A NEW VIEW OF THE PROBLEM

The best way to understand the challenge of weight loss and weight management is to look at the history of the problem. People often subscribe to the idea that you have a "start weight" and a "goal weight." In between those two numbers, you're "overweight." According to this idea, your problem is solved and disappears as soon as you reach your goal weight.

What's wrong with this approach? A lot. First of all, I feel that the word "overweight" doesn't really tell us much. It doesn't explain the situation, and it doesn't give us any direction in solving it.

The other problem with this approach is that it leaves out a crucial part of the solution: maintenance. News flash: *There's life after weight loss.* There really is. That's what weight management is all about. That's why the Structure House approach prepares you for it from the start. Our program provides you with numerous specific tools to help you keep the weight off and live with a mind-set that will ensure lifelong success.

Let's examine this situation a little more. I mentioned a moment ago that I don't like the word "overweight" because it doesn't tell us much, and it doesn't help us solve weight problems. Here's a better way of looking at this issue.

Imagine watching a videotape of your life. Mind you, this is a very special video. Every time you eat, the camera switches on and captures every calorie you consume. Can you imagine that? Here's what I think you'll do as you watch this dramatic miniseries.

You'll say, "Oh, look at this! The phone is ringing. I'm going into the kitchen to answer the phone. Now I'm talking to the caller. And while talking, I'm opening the refrigerator, I'm looking around in there, and I'm getting something to eat." Watching the video helps you add up all the calories you've consumed out of *habit*—automatic or ritualized eating that may evoke feelings of comfort and security.

You keep watching that videotape, and you say, "Now I'm watching a TV program, and I'm bored. Oh, look at this: that same old commercial is coming on again. I've seen it a zillion times. So I'm getting up, I'm going into the kitchen, I'm going to the refrigerator, and I'm getting a snack to eat." Before you know it, you've added up all the calories you've consumed out of *boredom*—filling up time or providing entertainment or stimulation.

As you continue to watch that videotape, you say, "Gosh, I remember that argument with my mother. I was so upset about all those things we said. Now look at that: I'm getting up, I'm going to the kitchen, I'm opening the fridge, and I'm getting something to eat." Before you know it, you can add up all the calories that you've consumed because of *stress*—a state of psychological or emotional imbalance.

Become the Director of Your Own Life's Video

There's no video-of-your-life technology, but at Structure House we have something that's even more powerful and effective. It's a better method of looking at this problem—a method that's more flexible and powerful than just thinking of the problem as "overweight." It's a method that doesn't just show you a number on a dial; it shows you your own behavior and how that behavior leads to weight gain. I'm talking about the Structure House Diary, a "device" that will give you a new view of the problem. The Diary will help you understand your relationship with food and shape it so you can eat to live, not live to eat. I'll explain the Diary in the next chapter.

STEP 6: MAINTAIN YOUR MOTIVATION

Do you like sports? Maybe, maybe not. But whether you do or don't, I'm sure you'll agree that a major part of playing any sport is motivation. In professional football, you need motivation to play a game that's aggressive, exhausting, and complex in its demands for stamina and teamwork. In professional golf, you need motivation to play for four long days without any team support. In Olympic gymnastics, you need motivation to maintain your precision and form. I could go on and on. Every sport demands its own kind of motivation.

What about the situation you're facing? Dealing with weight loss and weight maintenance isn't a sport, but it certainly requires motivation as great as—I'd say even greater than—what athletes have to muster. There are no time-outs, no halftime. You are in this game every hour of the day, every day of the week, every week of the year, every year of your life. Is it any wonder that your motivation is going to ebb and flow? Imagine a perpetual football game: you're on the field running the plays morning, noon, and night, day after day. It's not humanly possible. Imagine a perpetual golf game: you keep hitting that ball, looking for it, hitting it again, twenty-four hours a day. It couldn't be done. But dealing with weight loss and weight management is something you do 24/7.

So let's be realistic. Accept the fact that your motivation will ebb and flow. That's just part of the game. I urge you to be tolerant and gentle with your own ups and downs. You're taking responsibility and embracing change. These are wonderful, life-affirming steps! But you can't go full blast all the time. You need to find ways to pace yourself, coach yourself back into the game, and maintain your motivation.

Take a look at the word for a moment: *motivation*, the motive to action. When you break that word down, that's what that means—"a reason to act." Now, let me emphasize that you are capable of motivation. You know how I know that? Because you've had to take action simply to do what you're doing now. You've bought this book. Over the years, people have come to me and said, "I've been on more diets than I can count" or "I've tried every diet there is" or "I've done two dozen different diets." When they say that, they often feel they're being negative about themselves. But you know what I tell them? I say, "Good for you. All those different times you've said to yourself, 'I've had enough. I've got to do something about this,' you've been motivated to take action. Good for you."

What is motivation for weight loss? It comes in two forms. The first is physical: you don't feel so peppy, your clothes don't seem to fit, and your doctor says that you're close to becoming diabetic. Discomfort and worry prompt you to take action. What happens then? Well, it doesn't take much to improve your situation. If you lose even a small amount of weight, you'll start to regain your energy, you'll feel better, you'll look better, and your lab values will probably improve. I've had people come to me at Structure House after a fairly short period of time and say, "I feel like a million bucks. I haven't felt this great in ages." Well, if they feel like a million bucks, where is their physical motivation? It's gone, isn't it? What's going to tell them to move forward if they feel so good?

That's where the psychological issues come in: the price you pay— psychological pain. You look at yourself and say, "I'm not happy with how I feel about myself. I'm not having enough fun." Even if you feel better physically, the quality of your life may still be suffering. So you say, "I'm not satisfied." Is dissatisfaction a problem? I don't think so! Sometimes dissatisfaction creates a force that compels you to move forward.

How are we going to do that? Here's a suggestion that will help you— a way of coaching yourself back into the game.

The "Dear Me" Letter

I want you to write yourself a letter that will give you a sense of perspective in the future. I want you to write, "Dear Me: Here's what it's like to be me right now. Let me tell you how I'm not getting my needs met. Let me tell you how dissatisfied I am." I want you to capture everything you're feeling now so that you can read it in the future.

This letter is important, and I urge you to write it soon. Here's why. As soon as you begin to use the Structure House approach, you're going to start feeling better both physically and psychologically. That's great—it's what we want to happen. But once you begin to feel better, you'll start to forget your present dissatisfaction. After a while you may think, "Oh, it wasn't really so bad back then." You'll distance yourself from your own frustration in the past. I certainly understand how that can happen. But that attitude will be risky because it'll tend to undercut your motivation in the present. The "Dear Me" letter serves an important purpose by providing a kind of "before" photo that you can compare to what happens "after"—in the future. You'll be able to see in black and white what your situation was like. Rereading your "Dear Me" letter will help to give you a sense of context. It's essentially a letter from You-in-the-Past trying to help You-in-the-Present stay motivated as you undertake a crucial course of action.

Please write this letter! Reach into your heart and soul. Explain what you're going through and why you've decided to change your life. Dig deep into your feelings and experiences. Tell yourself in the bluntest possible terms how you feel and what you find frustrating about your life.

I want you to do more than just change your diet; I want you to change your life. Part of this change will happen because you'll change your relationship with food. And when you change your relationship with food, you alter what I call the equation of life. I want you to make food less attractive and less available. I want you to change so that life is more attractive and more available to you.

What follows are suggested themes for writing your "Dear Me" letter. The purpose of this exercise is to help you remember what inspired your desire to change. The letter needs to capture not only your *thoughts* about these issues but also your *feelings*. The "Dear Me" letter captures the root of your motivation—your reasons for wanting to Get Structured now and Stay Structured in the future.

Here are some themes that have showed up in Structure House participants' "Dear Me" letters and have given them a sense of perspective as they've used the Structure House approach:

HEALTH	SOCIAL	EMOTIONAL	ECONOMIC
Increased risk of illness	Reduced options for companionship	Low moods, risk of depression	Salary impairment
Achy joints and immobility	Dissatisfaction with appearance	Low self-esteem	Reduced options and discrimination
Sleep problems, including apnea	Hesitancy to go out	Anger and hostility	Increased cost of travel and clothing
Increased surgery risk	Negative reaction from others	Resentment	Time lost from work
Difficulty with hygiene	Options limited	Frustration	Increased food costs
Fatigue and shortness of breath	Isolation	Hopelessness	Inability to get insurance
Skin issues, including rashes	Reduced options for some activities	Anxiety and fear	Need for large car
Increased sweating	Reduced sexual ability	Shame and guilt	Increased medical costs

And here are some statements that Structure House participants have used in describing themselves in their "Dear Me" letters:

- "I get so out of breath more often."
- "My ankles hurt."
- "This weight problem causes my low back pain."
- "I have really bad abdominal cramping."
- "I can't play the sports I used to."
- "It's getting harder to find clothes that fit right."
- "Even expensive clothes don't look good on me."
- "Sometimes I think people are staring at me."
- "Wide shoes are hard to find."
- "I feel furious at myself when I overeat."
- "I get heartburn much more often now."

Now take some sheets of paper and write your own "Dear Me" letter.

CHANGE YOUR DIET—OR YOUR LIFE?

Life is a journey, and all journeys have a crossroads. For this journey, you reach the crossroads when you look and see one path that shows you the changes you need to make. That's daunting—I won't pretend otherwise. But the other path shows you what will happen if you *don't* make some changes. Looking at the need for change, you may say, "That looks hard! I'll have to change my life. I'm not so sure about this . . ." If that alternative looks worse to you, guess what you're going to do? You're going to choose *not* to change. You'll stay just where you are now. There's nothing so mysterious about that; it's just human nature.

If, on the other hand, you reach your crossroads and say, "That looks hard, but it looks better than the present!"—then guess what you're going to do? You're going to go seek that better place, you're going to feel compelled, motivated, and pushed to go forward, no question about that.

I'm sure you'll see the advantages of making a commitment. You have so much to gain. The Structure House approach offers you the opportunity to change not just your diet, but your life.

PART II

BE STRUCTURED

Implement the Behavioral Principles
of the Structure House
Weight Loss Plan

CHAPTER 4

Be Structured: Structured Eating and the Structure House Diary

"Getting Structured was marvelous. I listened to what they had to say at the beginning, and it sounded like something that was not radical. It was practical—based on real knowledge and experience."

—Arthur

"Getting Structured gave me a mind-set change. The most significant takeaway was being in control of the results."

—Melanie

"When I used the Structure House Diary regularly, I could see if a pattern was forming and work on it. For instance, there was a time I was so excited about going to an Indian restaurant that I turned around and drove home. I realized I was being controlled by food instead of the other way around. I went back to the restaurant another day, when I was calmer."

—Kate

The best way to create any change in your life—including change in your weight and your overall health—is through Structure. And by Structure I mean *a problem-solving strategy that you apply to the world around you to achieve an end result.* These words may seem odd when applied to a very personal, very human behavior like eating. But in fact, Structure *is* personal and it *is* human. Here's why.

All of us are born with a need for limits, direction, guidelines, and points of reference in our lives. Children, for instance, benefit from the structure that their parents provide, but even adults benefit from structure of many sorts—routines, societal expectations, rules, and laws. Imagine what driving would be like if we didn't have traffic rules. Imagine what communication would be like if we didn't have the structure of a vocabulary (agreement about what certain sounds mean) or the structure of grammar (agreement about how to assemble words into intelligible statements). Imagine what the world of work would be like if we didn't have agreed-upon assumptions about roles, tasks, schedules, and payment for services. In these and many other situations, we would all experience uncertainty and anxiety, and our interactions would degenerate into confusion, conflict, even chaos. Structure is a necessary part of every arena of our lives.

On a personal level, too, structure is crucial. The word "structure" may seem to imply *limits to what you can do,* and it does; however, structure also provides *situations that allow you to act in productive ways.* Structure provides you with freedom as well as limits. Because of structure, you aren't simply influenced by the forces of life; you can decide how to influence your environment in active ways.

For example, let's say that you feel unhappy about your current work situation. You decide that you need a new job. You could, of course, just go with the flow and hope that Fate intervenes. But to move forward more confidently and reliably on your career path, you're better off if you add Structure to your life by deciding what your goals are, how to achieve them, and which changes will make favorable outcomes more likely. You can also create Structure in your "project" of getting a new job by taking specific steps: updating your résumé, talking with a career counselor, getting organized to identify job opportunities, applying for new positions, and undergoing interviews. You could even have to take some adult ed classes to increase your job skills. In short, you don't let life simply act upon you; you act upon life. You do so by creating structure. Structure provides order, opportunities, and the possibility of change.

You may read what I'm telling you and object: "But sometimes don't events just *happen?*" Of course. Life is nothing if not unpredictable! But consider once again the issue of switching jobs. Perhaps you meet someone who just happens to need an employee with your qualifications. Or perhaps you chance upon a help-wanted ad for exactly the position you're looking for. Sheer luck isn't out of the question. But, as the saying goes, "Luck favors those who are well prepared." Structure is, among other things, a way of becoming well prepared. In the instance of an employment search, you're far more likely to find a new job *by creating the structure that will make certain events possible.* Precisely because life is filled with unpredictable events, Structure is useful—and often crucial—as a way of helping yourself cope with unpredictability. Ideally, building Structure into your life will help you shape reality to some extent and use it to your own advantage.

HOW DOES STRUCTURE APPLY TO WEIGHT AND HEALTH ISSUES?

Let's backtrack for a moment to our general definition: *Structure is a problem-solving strategy that we apply to the world around us to achieve an end result.* When applied to issues of weight and weight loss, I think we agree on the desired result: we want to lose weight, and we want to keep it off. No arguments there. But let's focus on a key part of the definition, the one that calls Structure "a problem-solving strategy." Suppose I gave you nothing more than a list of dos and don'ts about food. I tell you, "Eat Food Number 1. Eat Food Number 2. Eat Food Number 3," and so forth, one food after another. I also tell you, "Don't eat Food A. Don't eat Food B. Don't eat Food C," and so on, food after food. And I tell you lots of other dos and don'ts. Would that be a problem-solving strategy? No, not at all. It's little more than a shopping list—or a set of marching orders. We'd be here forever listing food after food after food, and this approach wouldn't really give you a set of tools to work with. Why is that a problem? Because you're going to encounter too many situations—and too *varied* a set of situations—to benefit sufficiently from an item-by-item list of dos and don'ts. But this item-by-item list is precisely what most diets provide, and it's one of the main reasons why diets usually fail.

Here's a better approach: let's survey the situation, come up with a true *strategy*, put that strategy into play, and see how it works out. Powerful problems need powerful strategies. We have a powerful problem here, right? So we need a powerful strategy. In the Structure House approach, that powerful strategy is called *Structured Eating.* Structured Eating gives you a flexible, effective approach to dealing with weight and health issues. You can adapt this strategy to your own situation as it develops over time and in many different settings.

WHAT IS STRUCTURED EATING?

Structured Eating is the eating you do each day to achieve two purposes: first, to nourish your body; and second, to maintain a desired level of weight. In practical terms, this means:

- Three nutritious meals a day consumed in appropriate portions
- No eating between meals
- No eating after dinner

These guidelines also mean an appropriate level of calories of balanced nutrition per day (determined on the basis of your sex, height, weight, medical condition, and age). This is food you *need* in order to stay alive, stay healthy, and achieve a desired level of weight.

Structured Eating Is More than *Just* Good Nutrition

The field of nutrition has done a fine job over the years of defining what our bodies require, so proper nourishment isn't hard to determine. How can we lose weight or attain a desired level of weight? That's primarily a matter of calculating the calories we take in and the calories we expend. Simply put: if you take in more calories than you expend, you'll gain weight; if you take in fewer calories than you expend, you'll lose weight.

But Structured Eating is more than just good nutrition. It's also a way of reaching two important insights:

Insight 1: *If Structured Eating is the eating you do each day to nourish your body and attain a desired level of weight, all the other eating you do is unnecessary for achieving these two goals.* This second kind of eating is Unstructured Eating. To put it another way: your body doesn't need more fuel than it requires for nutrition alone. Eating more food than you need is like overfilling your car's gas tank. Once you've filled the tank, it's full, right? The same thing holds true for your body. Once you've filled up your nutritional "gas tank," you don't need more fuel.

Insight 2: *Unstructured Eating will cause you to gain weight.* Why? Simply because the nutrition it provides will exceed what your body requires. If you continue to engage in too much Unstructured Eating, your caloric intake is certain to exceed your nutritional needs, and your body will store that extra nutrition as fat.

Structured Eating: A Strategy for Change

You have two basic choices for how to eat. Either you can *be in control of food*—or you can *let food control you*. Structured Eating is a way for you to be in control of food. By accepting that there are two fundamental kinds of eating, Structured Eating helps you reach insights about your relationship with food—not just what and when you eat but also *why* you eat. But these aren't just abstract insights! They have tangible, practical, day-to-day benefits. As a result of the insights you'll gain, you can:

- Isolate unhealthy kinds of eating
- Identify *antecedents*, or "eating triggers," that cause unhealthy eating to occur
- Learn where you need to make specific changes in your lifestyle, including changes that will help you establish a more balanced relationship with food

In short, Structured Eating is far more than just a diet. It's also a method of raising your consciousness about your habitual ways of eating. It's a way to change those habits and then establish new, better habits that work to your advantage. It's a specific, flexible set of tools that will help you change your life.

Acquiring and using these tools involves two steps.

Step 1: Accept that You Have an *Eating Problem*, Not a *Weight Problem*

Time after time, people tell me that they have a "weight problem." This perception gives rise to a huge misunderstanding that damages even the most earnest efforts toward weight loss and weight maintenance. If you make this same claim—"I have a weight problem"—I'd argue that, no, you don't have a weight problem at all; rather, you have an *eating problem*. Now say it to yourself: "I have an *eating problem*." See how different that feels? *Eating* is what you're doing that's problematic. *Weight* is only a result of the eating. You can't change the weight without changing the eating.

Most diets use only one measuring stick for progress: the scale. You go on the diet, you step on the scale, and you see if you've lost weight or gained weight. If you've lost weight, you're thrilled. If you've gained weight, you feel let down. The number on the dial is all that seems to matter.

This cycle of measurement sets you up for trouble. First of all, the scale doesn't tell the whole story. It focuses only on your weight, not on your behaviors that create the weight. Second, focusing on the scale simply substitutes one obsessive "high" for another. In the past, you got your "high" from food; now you're getting your "high" from weight loss. But the weight loss high is risky because it sets you up for disappointment. When your weight loss slows, your "high" bursts like a bubble. Here's the truth:

the scale doesn't really tell you enough about what you're doing, and it's not a good device for fostering change.

But if you don't use the scale as a measuring stick, how can you judge if you're doing well or poorly? My recommendation: judge yourself *by your behavior.* And to judge your behavior accurately, you need a better, more effective "device" for recording your actions, understanding the consequences of your actions, and choosing different actions in the future.

Step 2: Understand the Structure House Diary

The Structure House Diary is that device. It's a low-tech tool that is powerful not only by recording your eating behavior but also by helping to guide you toward change.

Now, I realize that as you read what I just told you, you may be thinking, "Great—another food diary! Just what I need!" Other weight loss plans certainly use food diaries. Perhaps you've used them yourself. Perhaps you've lost patience with food diaries!

Here's the truth, though: the Structure House Diary is different. It shows you not only *what* you eat but also *why* you eat. True, the Structure House Diary reveals the full range of your eating behaviors—not just meals but also the kinds of eating you do on the side (or on the sly!). But what's even more important, the Structure House Diary reveals the big picture for your eating: external and internal "events" (such as habit, boredom, and stress) that prompt Unstructured Eating in the first place. As a result, the Structure House Diary draws an important picture of your overall situation and your progress toward change much more accurately than simply noting what you've eaten. The detailed portrait it provides shows you the specific aspects of your lifestyle that will benefit from change.

The Structure House Diary is powerful and flexible in ways that go far beyond what other food diaries can accomplish. Here's why:

The Diary Lets You Structure One Day at a Time

You can't be aware of your eating behavior unless you track it. The Diary gives you a subtle but powerful tool to achieve that goal. But unlike the journals for other weight loss programs, the Structure House Diary lets you note not only *what you've eaten* but also *what you plan to eat*. That is, it structures future actions as well as recording present actions. You can see what a whole day's food will be before the day begins; then you can also track what you actually ate as the day took shape.

Why is this dual focus on the future and the present important?

First, because planning your meals will help you stay Structured. You can make thoughtful, imaginative choices in advance. Planning your meals and noting your plans in the Diary is a great way to choose healthier foods in appropriate quantities.

Second, this dual focus is important because it reveals many aspects of your behavior: patterns of eating, habits you weren't aware of, and connections between outside events at work, at home, and elsewhere that prompt Unstructured Eating.

The Diary Reveals Your Relationship with Food

By understanding not just *what* you eat when you are Structured but also *why* you eat when you are unstructured, the Diary reveals previously hidden aspects of your relationship with food. These are the behaviors that lead to weight gain. The insights you reach about your relationship with food will allow you to clarify what and how you need to change in your relationship with food. Since the Diary shows you the reasons for the "disconnect" between what you plan to eat and what you actually eat, you will gain a detailed portrait of which specific behaviors to change.

Suppose that you tend to eat a lot of chips or ice cream to "unwind" after work. You know that this behavior happens. But until you track your after-work snacks in the Diary, you probably won't realize *how often* it happens—or how much you actually eat each time you snack. This insight will be a breakthrough in its own right. Using the Diary also starts to reveal how you often nibble "on the sly" following, for example, arguments with your spouse or kids—another instance of using food to ease the tension you feel. The Diary gradually shows you how much you eat in response to stress. You hadn't noticed how often this happens—and you hadn't spotted the cause-effect relationship.

The Diary Gives You Goals to Aim For

Better yet, seeing the patterns in your eating allows you to plan goals for changes in your behavior, including how and what you eat. To continue the example of after-work snacking: you might plan alternative forms of stress relief, such as going for a walk once you get home, listening to a favorite music CD, or putting on an exercise DVD and doing an aerobic workout to let off some steam. As you explore these options and note your activities, the Diary will also show you how close you've come to the goals you've set. Once you've reached your goals, the Diary gives you a sense of accomplishment for having completed what you set out to do.

The Diary Presents You with Options for Manageable Change

Rather than putting you in a position of striving for huge, ever-escalating goals, the Diary allows you to achieve steady, incremental progress that will add up more effectively in the long run. Using the Diary provides insights that will accumulate day after day. You can plan your responses, too, and build on them over time.

Let me ask you a question: How much do you really eat? If you're like most people, you don't actually know. Do you keep track of your portions at mealtimes? Do you note when you snack—and how much? When you cook meals, do you ever sneak more than just a taste of what you're cooking? And when you're cleaning up after dinner, do you eat even more while you throw out the leftovers? Well, maybe you have a fail-safe memory of all the food you eat. Or perhaps you have "hard numbers" because you count calories. But that's still not much information to work with, is it? And even if you have a pretty good idea of how much you eat, you probably don't have a clear sense of the cause-effect circumstances that influence your eating. You probably aren't entirely aware of the external events or the internal feelings that prompt you to eat in the ways you do. And because you're not clear about many of these issues, it's difficult for you to take hold of the situation and change the aspects of your behavior that are causing you some frustration.

But the Structure House Diary offers you a way out of this dilemma. How? By helping you answer these crucial questions:

- What events prompt you to eat more than usual?
- What emotions prompt you to eat more than usual?
- What events disrupt your good intentions to regulate your eating?
- What people around you may tempt you to eat more or less?

- What other events, emotions, or people have influence on how, when, and why you eat?

Answering these questions over time tells you what you're doing. It also helps you make the necessary changes to your behavior. And if you can change your behavior, many of your feelings and attitudes will also change. These changes, in turn, will further change your behavior. And more changes to your behavior will further change your feelings and attitudes. The vicious cycle that I described earlier—the cycle that makes weight loss and health issues so difficult—will be replaced by a positive, creative cycle of change and personal growth.

"Why Can't I Just Count Calories?"

As you read my explanation, you may protest: "This is too complicated. Why can't I just count calories? Won't *that* lead to change?"

I mentioned earlier that all behavior, including eating, takes place within a context, an environment. Calories alone don't tell you much about the environments that influence your eating: who you're with (friends, family, coworkers), what's going on around you (a party, an outing), and how you're feeling (bored, happy, sad, anxious). To understand your eating, you need to understand far more than just the number of calories you're consuming. And you need far more than a calorie count if you want to foster change.

Consider these two scenarios:

Scenario 1. Let's say that on a given day you're not dieting. That evening, you decide to watch TV. There's not much on the tube that interests you, however, so you feel bored. Then a commercial comes on for Duncan Hines. You see a beautiful cake, complete with swirly icing, and it sure looks good! Your response: you decide to get some leftover cake from your refrigerator. You get up, walk to the refrigerator, open the door, and reach in with your hand. You feel the cool air on your hand, you pull the cake out, and then you feel the warm air. You go to the drawer and get a fork. You cut and eat your cake. Tasty! You return to your chair and watch the program—which is still boring!

Scenario 2. But let's say you've decided to begin a diet that substitutes low-calorie foods for high-calorie foods. What happens? That evening you decide to watch TV.

There's not much on that interests you, however, and you're bored. Then a commercial comes on for Duncan Hines. You see a beautiful cake, complete with swirly icing, and it sure looks good! Your response: you decide to get some leftover cake from your refrigerator. But then you remember your diet and how it substitutes low-calorie foods for high-calorie foods. So instead of taking some cake, you decide to eat a carrot. You get up, walk to the refrigerator, open the door, and put your hand in. You feel the cool air on your hand, you pull the carrot out, and then you feel the warm air. You go to the drawer, get a knife, cut the carrot, and eat it. It's not as tasty as cake! So you return to the chair and watch the program—which is still boring. And you're still thinking about the cake.

Now tell me honestly: what has changed from Scenario 1 to Scenario 2? Not much. If you can think of your behavior as a chain of discrete actions, Scenario 2 differs from Scenario 1 only because you've taken out a single link—a piece of cake—and you've substituted another link—a carrot. That's all. You've simply switched one food for another.

What would be a better approach for fostering change? If you want *real* change, you have to create a different behavior *at the first link*, not just at a later link way down the chain. And to create a different behavior, you need to understand your old behavior: the link between *what you're feeling* and *how that feeling prompts you to eat.* In short, you need to understand what triggers your eating.

WHY THE STRUCTURE HOUSE DIARY IS SO POWERFUL: UNDERSTANDING ANTECEDENTS—YOUR "EATING TRIGGERS"

By now I hope you've accepted the reality that *food* isn't your problem. The problem is *what you do with food*—how you use it, when, and why. It's your behavior toward food that leads to overeating, which in turn leads to weight gain. For this reason, one of the most crucial tasks before you in gaining control of your weight and weight-related issues is to understand *what your behaviors are in relation to food* and *why you use food in nonnutritional ways.*

So here's my question: If you recognize that your eating behavior is the core of your weight problem, how can you zero in on problematic behaviors, identify them, and change them?

I've stated that the best way to answer that question is to track the situation in your Structure House Diary. This process will allow you to see the reasons for your Unstructured Eating. At Structure House, we call those reasons *antecedents*. Antecedents are the hidden "eating triggers" that prompt you to eat for nonnutritional reasons. Understanding your antecedents will clarify why you use food as you do—and then provide you with specific options for change. The concept of antecedents is why both the Structured Eating strategy—and the Structure House Diary as the "engine" for driving that strategy—are so powerful.

The Power of Taking Small Steps

I believe that we all have the greatest chance of success when change happens in small steps. Global efforts to change are bound to fail. So if global efforts won't work, what will? You may remember a movie some years back called *What About Bob?* Bill Murray starred as a wacky patient, and Richard Dreyfuss played his therapist. Bill Murray went to his therapist and asked, "How do I change?" The doctor replied, "You take baby steps, baby steps." So the entire movie was about Bill Murray trying to take baby steps to change. Well, that's correct—baby steps are what help you change. And determining the antecedents of your actions will help you find the baby steps that lead to making big changes.

For example, let's say that you love going to the movies, but you're aware that you always eat popcorn at the theater, one of those big buckets—a habit that contributes to your weight. You know that you somehow need to eliminate this type of Unstructured Eating. Now, you could certainly respond in a global way to this issue and say, "Well, the solution is simple. For the rest of my days, I'll never, ever go to the movies." But that's the global approach—one that's too drastic, too all-or-nothing—and it won't work. Instead, it's better to find the small steps you can take with this scenario.

What are the antecedents that are necessary for you to eat popcorn at the movies?

- You need time to go to the movies.
- You need a movie to go see.
- You need transportation to get to the theater.
- You need money to buy the ticket for the movie you're going to see.
- Finally, you need money to buy the popcorn once you're in the theater.

Instead of making a drastic, global response to this type of unstructured eating—depriving yourself forever of going to the movies—why not take a smaller, more effective step? How about if you take *only enough money to buy the ticket for the movie*? Once you're inside the theater, you'll have no money left to buy popcorn, so there will be no popcorn. You've made just a small step, but you've obtained the result you're looking for.

By approaching change in this way—by looking for antecedents and for small steps to take in response to the antecedents—you can begin to make better headway in changing your eating habits.

Listening to the scenario I've described, you may say, "Well, that's just fine when it's a simple situation like going to the movies. But aren't most situations more complicated than that?" You may worry that the scenarios you face involve many more antecedents—perhaps an unmanageable number.

Well, then, let me ask you this question: how many antecedents do you think you're going to discover by keeping a Structure House Diary? Twenty? Fifteen? Ten? Five?

No—just three!

Here are the three antecedents you're going to discover for all of your Unstructured Eating:

- Antecedent 1: Habit
- Antecedent 2: Boredom
- Antecedent 3: Stress

That's it. Just three. Let's explore them one by one.

Antecedent 1: Habit

Habits are *automatic or ritualized behavior that can evoke feelings of comfort and security.* A habit may involve "going through the motions" in ways that seem to make no sense or have no content; on the other hand, habit often has a hidden agenda, some sort of underlying emotional state that you may not even recognize. For instance, a seemingly content-free habit of eating a big dish of ice cream after work may, in fact, be your way of releasing pent-up frustration after a day of conflict or uncertainty at work.

Let's face it, we're all creatures of habit. Putting on your garments in a particular sequence is a habit. Tapping your toe to music is a habit. Cleaning up your kitchen in a recurrent sequence of steps is a habit. And all of us develop food habits, too. Putting extra butter on mashed potatoes is a habit. Eating a snack on arriving home after work is a habit. Munching on pretzels while watching TV is a habit. Going to the kitchen for seconds—or thirds—is a habit. Individually, these habits aren't necessarily a problem. But if you accumulate enough food habits, you'll start accumulating weight as well. Thin people can develop food habits, too. You just happen to have more food habits than thin people because of your rich learning history with food.

Everything in the Structure House program is designed to help you start changing habits. How? By using the Structure House Diary to become aware of them. By helping you understand how ordinary habits are the antecedents of much of your eating behavior. By helping you substitute other, more constructive behaviors for Unstructured Eating.

Antecedent 2: Boredom

Boredom—a lack of gratification or reinforcement—is your second antecedent of eating. Boredom can result from the absence of enjoyment, gratification, or positive reinforcement. It's often the result of an inability to get your needs met. Ideally, you have a lifestyle that provides stimulation and satisfaction. If it doesn't, you may tend to use food to fill up time, provide entertainment, or create a sense of stimulation. You have nothing else to do, so you eat. Yet boredom, too, may express far more than what's on the surface. Eating out of boredom may be a way to cope with loneliness and hurt, or a way to distract yourself from a sense of frustration or emptiness.

Boredom can also become part of a cycle of antecedents and problematic behaviors. As you gain weight, you tend to stop doing things. You cut back on activities because you feel awkward, uncomfortable, or embarrassed. And when you cut back on activities, there's less to do, which easily leads to boredom. But boredom is like a vacuum. There's less going on, less to do, less to think about—so, in that state of mind, you look around for something to do. Guess what you often see around you? Food. Food is readily available, inexpensive, and user-friendly. You don't need to get dressed for it, make reservations for it, or even have company to enjoy it. Some of your best eating has been done alone, right?

When it comes to changing boredom, I want to ask you two questions that are critical to this task. First, how do you spend your time—all twenty-four hours? And second, are you spending your twenty-four hours in ways that please you? If the answer is no, you have some lifestyle work to do. But the Structure House Diary will help you get a handle on boredom, and it will help to limit the ability of boredom to cause Unstructured Eating. (Chapter 10 also offers specific, detailed steps you can take to explore a more creative lifestyle.)

Antecedent 3: Stress

Finally, there's stress, a state of psychological imbalance. When many people feel stressed, they eat. This cause-effect relationship happens not only in response to "bad stress" (work hassles, marital conflicts, financial pressures, and so forth) but also in reaction to "good stress" (a promotion, a purchase of a new house, the birth of a child, the birth of a grandchild)—anything that throws you out of your normal equilibrium. When you're coping with stress, food can be tempting to use as a tranquilizer or sedative. It quiets your nerves. But as an antecedent to eating, stress can cause a lot of problems. "Self-medicating" stress with Unstructured Eating can cause weight gain and aggravate weight-related health problems. In all of these situations, it's better to pinpoint the stresses you're experiencing and to understand how they prompt Unstructured Eating. Later chapters of this book will include information on stress management, relaxation, and other ways to cope with stress.

Think about all the different kinds of stress that can prompt Unstructured Eating:

Negative Emotional States:

- "I'm so furious about how my boss scolded me in front of everyone."
- "I'm angry—but I can't risk venting what I feel."
- "I'm so depressed [anxious, frustrated, guilty]."
- "I feel so helpless."
- "I'm so lonely."

Negative Physical States:

- "I feel really shaky."
- "I think I'm sick."
- "Gosh, I'm so exhausted."
- "I have so many aches and pains."
- "I can't seem to get to sleep."

Positive Emotional States (related to self):

- "I'm feeling happy about myself."
- "I feel excited about what happened [or what's going to happen]."
- "It's so great that I've been able to [achieve success at something]."

Testing Personal Control:

- "I wanted to see if I could use food in moderation."
- "I wanted to see if I could be around my eating buddy without eating, too."

Urges and Temptations:

- "I began to think about how good it would be to eat."
- "There was food in the house—I just couldn't help having some of it."
- "I was at the party, and everyone else was eating."

Interpersonal Conflict:

- "My husband [or wife] and I weren't getting along."
- "My kids were driving me crazy."
- "I needed to get up the courage to face up to my boss [relative, friend, whomever] before we started our confrontation [argument, discussion]."
- "People reject me [or don't seem to like me]."

Social Pressure:
- "I was at the dinner party [barbecue, picnic, whatever], and there was so much food around, and everyone else was eating."
- "It seemed impolite to refuse the food they offered me."

Positive Emotional States (related to others):
- "I wanted to help celebrate at the birthday party [wedding, Bar Mitzvah, whatever] along with everyone else."
- "I felt close to him [her] on our date, and the food was part of what made being there so special."

The Most Important Single Step . . .

Why are habit, boredom, and stress so important? And why is tracking these antecedents important, too? I assure you it's not just accountancy. The reason: tracking this information lets you use the Structure House Diary as a self-evaluation tool. By identifying your antecedents, you learn why you eat. Noting your antecedents over time will reveal important patterns, and the insights you gain will allow you to change. If you don't identify your antecedents, you'll never know what behaviors to change. *The most important single commitment you can make in the Structure House program is to continue tracking your antecedents.* Then you can look more deeply into what the antecedents mean. You will grasp the true cause-effect relationship between your antecedents and your Unstructured Eating. You can start to see these antecedents not just as *external events or circumstances* but as *internal emotional states.*

Here's an example.

Let's say that you go to work and your boss gets angry at you. You feel bad about this outburst, so you retreat and eat a whole bag of cookies. Later, you note the incident in your Structure House Diary and write the word "stress" on today's page. What I want you to realize, however, is that the antecedent wasn't *the interaction with your boss.* The antecedent was *whatever internal reaction you felt as a result of the interaction with your boss.* To put it another way: the antecedent is the emotional resonance—anger, humiliation, frustration, whatever—to the external incident. Perhaps you have poor self-esteem or you're afraid that you're "not good enough." Perhaps you're scared of rejection or conflict. Perhaps you're worried about your anger toward your boss. All of those antecedents can be activated by the situation I've described.

Why is labeling antecedents so important? It's important in the same way that labeling the circuit breakers in your household electrical panel is important. If the lights go out in the dining room, you need to know which switch to flip to turn the power back on. If you have an urge or a craving for food, you need to go through your little internal electrical panel to figure out what switch got flipped there. Knowing how these "connections" work will save you a lot of trouble. If your boss gets angry in the future, you can tell yourself, "I get upset because I'm hungry for approval [or whatever prompts your anger]. Feeding that hunger by eating all those cookies won't solve anything—and it'll backfire anyway. So I won't eat like that when my boss chews me out. I'll figure out some other way to deal with my frustration."

Looking more deeply at antecedents is, ultimately, the key to change. Why? For these reasons:

- By understanding antecedents, you will understand what's prompting your Unstructured Eating.
- When you understand what's prompting your Unstructured Eating, you can zero in on emotional states or beliefs and start to change them.
- By changing them, you will gain control over your choices—including the choices of what, when, and under what circumstances you should eat.

Which brings us back to the practical, powerful, nuts-and-bolts tool for Structured Eating: the Structure House Diary.

HOW TO USE THE STRUCTURE HOUSE DIARY AS A LONG-TERM STRATEGY FOR CHANGE

How can you achieve change? By using the Structure House Diary to track your eating and set specific goals for yourself. The Diary is your commitment to change. You can't be aware of what you do with food unless you track it. The Diary allows you to structure one day at a time, which in turn lets you shape your behavior by taking specific, small steps that will add up quickly for both immediate and long-term benefit. Your Structure House Diary tells you how much you're eating, what environmental changes you have to make, what your Structured Eating goal is, and what you do with your time.

The central task in Getting Structured is the daily use of the Structure House Diary. By recording your preplanned Structured Eating, your activities, your Unstructured Eating, and your antecedents, you'll gain a clearer and clearer picture over time of what and why you eat. The process of clarifying this picture will become a source of positive energy to change your lifestyle, lose weight, and improve your overall health.

Let's walk through a typical day and see how you'll use the Structure House Diary.

Below is an example of a two-page (left and right) diary entry. Food is structured for Breakfast (BF), Lunch (L), and Dinner (D).

The Structure House Diary

The Left-Hand Page

Structured Eating (SE) is the three meals you eat each day to meet your nutritional requirements. You plan these meals in advance and note them in your Structure House Diary; you also specify your planned activities for each day.

Date: October 17 _____   Weight: 197 _____

Structured Eating

Meal	Place
BF:	Kitchen
2 slices French toast	200
1 cup strawberries	50
½ cup yogurt	50
1 tablespoon low-calorie syrup	10

310 c   (c = calories)

L: Restaurant
Wendy's grilled chicken   200
Salad without dressing   80

                                                  280c

D: Dining Room
3-ounce sirloin steak   180
1 baked potato   160
½ cup green beans   15
3-ounce salad with 1 ounce low-calorie dressing   40
½ cup melon   25

                                                  420 c

                                    SE total   1,010 c

If you maintained Structured Eating, you would note your activities on the left-hand column of the page below, but you wouldn't note any antecedents, since those apply only to Unstructured Eating.

The Right-Hand Page

Time: In this column you plan and record your use of time during the day. Plan your work activities, commitments, and exercise; record your times and activities. Take control of your time. Reward yourself in ways other than by eating. If you don't select interesting, varied activities, they probably won't happen.

Unstructured Eating (USE): USE is any and all eating you do other than the three preplanned meals. Record USE in the antecedents column. Describe the food and calories. Write USE next to the activities to which it is related—for instance, "Errands—USE." Then give details, such as "Bought doughnuts while shopping."

Antecedents: Note the hidden "eating triggers" that led to your Unstructured Eating.

Time/USE		Antecedents
6–8 A.M.	Shower, dress	
8–10 A.M.	BF, walk, clean	
10 A.M.–12 noon	errands	
12 noon–2 P.M.	lunch/Sally	
2–4 P.M.	Car pool	
4–6 P.M.	Relax, phone, fix dinner	
6–8 P.M.	Dinner, change clothes	
8–10 P.M.	Movie	
10–12 midnight	get ready for bed	
12 midnight–6 A.M.	sleep	

USE total   c [c = calories]

SE total   1,010 c

Each of your diary pages can be different, but every one will provide a goal for tomorrow—one very small, achievable step at a time.

When you enter information in your diary:

- Remember what you have learned about nutrition to structure your eating, and
- Remember what you have learned about your needs, how to get them met, and how to structure your time.

Now let's suppose that on the same day we noted earlier, you ended up changing your activities—and the meals you'd planned—at the last moment. In short, you were Unstructured. The left-hand page of your Diary would look the same as before, since it indicates the Structure you planned before the day began. The right-hand page, however, would look like this—with added data for Unstructured Eating and the antecedents (habit, stress, and boredom) that preceded it.

Time/USE		Antecedents	
6–8 A.M.	Shower, dress	Got up late, rushed—stress	Event 1
8–10 A.M.	Skip BF		
10 A.M.–12 noon	Errands		
12 noon–2 P.M.	Lunch/Sally	Temptation of deli; Ate cheese steak, fries, jumbo Coke—habit/stress	Event 2
2–4 P.M.	Car pool		
4–6 P.M.	Relax, phone, fix dinner	Argument with friend; changed dinner plans— stress	Event 3
6–8 P.M.	Dinner, change clothes		
8–10 P.M.	Movie		
10–12 midnight	Get ready for bed	Friends stayed and brought snacks; ate chips and dip—habit	Event 4
12 midnight–6 A.M.	Sleep		

USE total   USE total 1,660 c (c = calories)

SE total   Day total 1,660 c

Now, what can this Diary entry tell you? Plenty! Here is an example of what you would find if you reviewed your Diary. Let's look at each change.

Event 1: You Skipped Breakfast

There may be various explanations here, so let's examine two of them.

- **Explanation 1:** You overslept and got up too late to eat before racing off to work. Well, oversleeping can certainly happen. Don't worry about skipping breakfast, as long as it doesn't happen too often. There's a legitimate concern, though, if skipping breakfast is a frequent occurence—particularly if this behavior is part of your historical eating pattern that has led to excess weight.

- **Explanation 2:** You just didn't feel like eating breakfast. This can be a more serious issue. Skipping breakfast can suggest a major unraveling of Structured habits. Why does it cause so much concern? Because it suggests that you're going back to the old habits that led to your weight gain in the first place. If you're reverting to old habits, you face a serious problem, and you should take steps to correct the situation as soon as possible. What sorts of steps? One of the best is to do a "Structure House Day" at home. Plan an entire day that will be your special day. To the greatest degree possible, clear the deck of responsibilities and obligations. Structure three meals. Know what you are going to eat and where. Make a plan for exercise during that day, too. Structure your time to take care of yourself. Reread sections of this book to reinforce what you've learned. Finally, review your Diary to look for clues for why you might be backing off from Structure. The clues are there. Perhaps your days are becoming increasingly Unstructured. Perhaps your stress has increased to levels that historically have led to your Unstructured Eating.

Event 2: You Changed Your Plans for Lunch

We need to ask an additional question here: Were you Structured for the food you ate in your new lunch selection?

- **Explanation 1:** "Yes, I was Structured, but a situation came up that changed my plans." Another way to respond is "Yes. A situation came up that I felt was unavoidable and changed my plans. Nevertheless, I was Structured." This sort of event will happen from time to time. You responded to the new situation but did a good job of staying Structured.

- **Explanation 2:** "No, I wasn't Structured because people showed up and invited me out unexpectedly." This can be serious—it could be one of the early warning signs of unraveling Structure. Ask yourself: *Are the people who showed up and/or the situations they present common challenges to my staying Structured?* If yes, you may need to take steps to regain control of the situation. Don't necessarily expect to regain control of every situation you find yourself in. What is important is learning from the situation so you can prevent a repeat in the future. Look at the people who showed up. Do they do this often? Are they "eating buddies" who encourage Unstructured Eating? If so, you will have to deal with them the next time they call. You need to set boundaries for what you're willing to do. On the other hand, this situation may occur only once in a while. If so, it doesn't necessarily mean that your Structure is unraveling.

- **Explanation 3:** "No, I wasn't Structured because I didn't feel like ordering the food I'd Structured beforehand. I felt like eating something I used to eat." If this is the reason, it can be a serious problem. How frequent is this behavior? If it doesn't happen very often, it may be okay. This sort of thing happens to all of us. If it's frequent, however, it's definitely a warning sign. It is warning you that your Structure is about to become totally unraveled. This would especially be the case if this kind of Unstructured Eating is part of your historical pattern. Go back through your Diary to look for other episodes of Unstructured Eating. Is there a pattern in your Unstructured Eating? If so, this is often a sign of unmet needs. You may, for the first time, be able to identify your true needs by reviewing your Diary. Are you getting enough sleep? Are you exercising enough? Are you doing enough for yourself? Are you allowing stress to increase without taking care of yourself?

- **Explanation 4:** "I was Unstructured because I was upset." This too would be a serious situation. In response, you should note the source of tension. Doing so is very important, as what you're noting may indicate an area that requires change. Perhaps you are just doing too much each day. You aren't taking care of yourself. You have stopped exercising, which means you're missing out on a great source of stress reduction. You aren't spending enough time with people or activities that you find fulfilling.

Event 3: You Changed Your Plans for Dinner

Why? And—this follow-up question is important—did you substitute Structured foods? Here are four explanations:

- **Explanation 1:** "Yes, I substituted Structured foods." Don't worry as long as substitutions aren't something you do too frequently. Be honest with yourself as to the frequency of these events. Your Diary should reflect the reality of what you're doing.

- **Explanation 2:** "I was Unstructured at dinner because I got upset." Again, note the source of tension.

- **Explanation 3:** "I don't know. I just grabbed the first available thing!" If this happens, ask yourself whether your environment was Unstructured. If so, change your environment by eliminating Unstructured foods—get them out of your fridge and your cupboards, don't buy them when you go shopping, and so forth. Otherwise, the presence of Unstructured foods will be a repeated source of Unstructured Eating.

- **Explanation 4:** "I ate because I felt bored." In this case, look for ways to increase your source of satisfaction and reinforcement. Missing opportunities to Structure your time will cause you a lot of problems. Make certain that you have Structured your time ahead of time. If time is left Unstructured, and if you historically filled your empty time with food, you will do so in the future.

Event 4: You Were Unstructured and Really, Really Ate Too Much

Once again, it's important to ask *Why?* We also need to ask how often you do this. The two likeliest explanations:

- **Explanation 1:** "I don't often find myself changing my plans. This is really unusual." If that's your explanation, don't worry. This is not a problem.

- **Explanation 2:** "I change my plans frequently." This answer suggests a problem in how you're planning events. It's possible that you're selecting activities that aren't really of interest to you and that don't fulfill your needs. You should reexamine your schedule.

As before, the crucial question is *Why?* But it's equally crucial to ask, *Did your Unstructured behavior involve other people?* Consider these explanations:

- **Explanation 3:** "My behavior did involve other people." If Unstructured Eating involves certain people and the behavior is frequent, you should examine your contact with these people. You may need to assert yourself in that situation. What to do? Assert yourself in advance. Set guidelines with them. Speak with them so that the guidelines are clear. Remember, you have a right to do what you need to!

- **Explanation 4:** "No, people weren't an issue." If certain situations or circumstances are a problem for you, examine the reasons you find yourself in these situations. You may need to make some changes. Perhaps you have developed a series of activities over the years that really aren't very rewarding or enjoyable. Or else you bunch together a series of activities that just create tension for you. Remember, balance is essential in leading a life without Unstructured Eating. Yes, you have activities that are obligations and duties—fair enough. But you should balance them throughout any given day with activities that are "want-tos," not "ought-tos."

These examples should give you some initial insights into understanding how Unstructured behavior—whether related to food or time—comes about. In particular, notice how Events 3 and 4 are part of one larger complex. Following the argument with your friend, you changed your dinner plans, which was a problem in its own right. But your state of feeling upset and wanting to comfort yourself then led to more Unstructured Eating when other friends showed up late with snacks. Often an event has more than one subevent as a component. However, each event needs to be examined independently. Remember, Structure gives you a target to aim for as you decide upon your behaviors. Structure is measurable, and it goes by one act, one day at a time. How you respond is your own decision.

Here are two blank Structure House Diary pages that you can photocopy for your own use. You can also find and download these pages from the Structure House Web site at: www.structurehouse.com.

Date: _____   Weight: _____

Structured Eating
Meal   **Place**
BF:

_____
                                                          c

_____

L:

_____
                                                          c
_____

D:

_____
                                                          c
_____

_____

SE total   c

_____

Time/USE	Antecedents
6–8 A.M.	
8–10 A.M.	
10–12 NOON	
12–2 P.M.	
2–4 P.M.	
4–6 P.M.	
6–8 P.M.	
8–10 P.M.	
10–12 MIDNIGHT	
12 MIDNIGNT–6 A.M.	

USE total   c

Day total   c

THE CHALLENGE AND THE OPPORTUNITY: DEAL WITH UNSTRUCTURED EATING

Remember, Getting Structured is a combination of Structured Eating, using the Structure House Diary, and tracking the eating behaviors caused by three antecedents (habit, boredom, and stress). This is a process, not a quick fix that occurs overnight. It's a set of behaviors that you need to practice over a period of time. But it's accessible and effective in helping you change what may be years of ingrained eating patterns. But you may ask, "What if I can't stay Structured all the time? What if I revert to Unstructured Eating?"

Think of it this way: Unstructured Eating is going to happen. I guarantee it. There *will* be times when all your best efforts to stay Structured just don't work out. But that's okay. It's part of the process.

So if it's inevitable, should you *plan* Unstructured Eating? No, never. Why? Because you don't need to—it'll happen all by itself! But don't get upset when it does. Just get back to Structure with your very next meal. Unstructured Eating isn't a disaster; in fact, it's helpful because it reveals the hidden reasons behind your eating—showing you what your relationship with food is, why food is so important to you. It shows you the antecedents. And it suggests new ways for you to change.

Once you accept that Unstructured Eating is a part of your reality, here's a sequence of steps you should follow whenever you consider doing it.

- Never say to yourself, "I can't eat that." In fact, you can eat whatever you want!

- *Before* you go ahead and eat in an Unstructured way, determine the antecedent of your eating. The time *before* you eat is crucial to the process of learning *why* you eat. It's a moment that you must learn to freeze, because once you start to eat, you stop thinking; you are unable to think.

- Decide how to deal with the antecedent you've identified; then act on your decision.

- If you still want to eat, put one or more of the following "obstacles" (labeled **"TAD"**) between *your thought about eating* and *the act of eating:*

- **T**ime (delay at least 25 to 30 minutes)
- **A**ctivity (go for a walk, do some other sort of exercise, start a conversation, do an enjoyable activity, etc.)
- **D**istance (go to a place where there is no food available)

- Remember, when you eat, you're making a statement: "Eating is the best thing in this whole world that I can do for myself at this time." Your goal is to figure out some other action that's more constructive, more helpful, and more satisfying in the long run.

In short, Unstructured Eating provides both a challenge and an opportunity. Every time you consider the option of Unstructured Eating, you're faced with the challenge of whether you can decide not to eat in a way that may work against your best interests. At the same time, you have an opportunity to examine *why* you eat more closely and then take better control of your choices.

But maybe you'll respond to the challenge and the opportunity with defiance. You'll say, "I don't really need to keep that diary! I don't need to plan my meals ahead of time! I don't need to do all this stuff!"

Or maybe you'll say, "Look, I want something that works fast. I want to go 'cold turkey' and shake these weight issues once and for all."

Here's how I'd respond. It's true that some weight loss programs have borrowed methodology from drug and alcohol treatment programs. In certain fasting methods of weight loss, for instance, you just don't eat. But here's the catch: There are major differences between treating drug or alcohol abuse and treating weight issues. For drugs and alcohol, the treatment of choice is to go cold turkey. You abstain totally: no drugs, no alcohol. Well, you can certainly go cold turkey with drugs or alcohol because your body doesn't need those substances to survive. But that's not true regarding food. Sooner or later, you have to go back to eating. That's just reality, folks.

So here's how I see the situation: *You can't live without food.* In one way or another, you're going to need food for the rest of your life. Structured Eating is the way to live with food. Is it challenging? For some people, it is; for others, not so much. It does, in fact, require that you do change a number of your ideas and a number of your behaviors. Is it painful? Well, change can be painful. But so is excess weight. So is feeling that you don't look as attractive as you could. So is feeling that your social life has deteriorated. So is reluctance to exercise, to be fit, to enjoy all the activities that you may have abandoned. So is learning that you have high blood pressure, joint pains, elevated blood sugar, shortness of breath, and cardiac problems.

Here's the truth: With pain, you change. If you feel comfortable, you won't change. That's just human nature. What isn't working in your life? What is painful in your life? Look in the mirror. What you see there says that you're using food in problematic ways. You say you don't like that picture. Why is there a difference between what you see and what you want to see?

With courage, you can meet the challenge and take charge of an opportunity.

The Structure House approach is flexible, portable, and adaptable. It's a tool kit for change. Structured Eating is the "kit," and inside the kit are many separate tools, including the Structure House Diary. The rest of this book will give you other tools. Now take them, use them, and make changes to your life.

CHAPTER 5

Be Structured at Home: Eating Well and Losing Weight in Your Own Kitchen

"Don't keep junk food in the house. If your husband or children need that food, either put it in a special off-limits area or ask them to keep it somewhere out of your sight. If it's in the house, you're going to want to eat it."

—Anella

"When you have had enough to eat, cover your plate with a napkin; it helps to keep you from nibbling and picking. Don't douse your foods with condiments; that only hides the true flavor. Snacking may work for some people, but not for me—I don't know when to stop."

—Sandra

"I used to have many more activities centered around food, so all of that has changed. When we have dinner parties [now], we have healthy food. A lot of my friends,

they've been thrilled, because that's how they wanted to
eat anyway."

—Genelle

We live in an age of mind-boggling abundance. American supermarkets are full of beautiful produce, high-quality meats and fish, baked goods of every kind, exotic food specialties from around the world, and processed foods of such vast variety that it often induces "choice fatigue." No matter what your tastes or whims, you can purchase whatever you want. And with American kitchens increasingly well equipped and sophisticated, you can prepare your meals exactly to your taste. These aspects of contemporary American life are a big boost in efforts to stay Structured. That's the good news.

The bad news? We're all just about drowning in food! With so much food so readily available, it's easy to get Unstructured, overeat, and suffer the consequences. American supermarkets are a marvel—but they offer marvelous opportunities for nutritional trouble. The familiarity and comfort of your own kitchen offer flexibility and convenience, but they also challenge you with many temptations that complicate the task of staying Structured. The privacy of home makes it easy to fall prey to habit, boredom, and stress.

How can you manage this situation? I've helped many Structure House participants cope creatively with these issues. In this chapter, I'll provide you with a multitude of ideas for staying Structured at home. Upcoming chapters will offer the tools you need to stay Structured at the supermarket, in restaurants, and while traveling.

TASK 1: UNDERSTAND YOUR FOOD ENVIRONMENT—AND BUST THE BAD HABITS IT CREATES

Your food environment consists of all the places around you that affect how you obtain, prepare, and eat food. It certainly includes your home, but it also includes your workplace, your car, your local grocery store, and the restaurants you visit. Your food environment includes many positive features, but it also sets up all sorts of challenges: distractions from your menu plans, temptations to snack, and opportunities for Unstructured Eating. Friends arrive with gifts of food. The TV, magazines, the Web, and the newspaper all show you tempting treats. So many voices tell you to *Eat, eat, eat* that it's easy to forget your best intentions and abandon your best-laid plans. But if you can understand your food environment—and see how it affects your eating habits—you're already ahead of the game.

Habit Busters: A Key to Structure

Does your food environment create some bad eating habits? Probably— it's true for almost everyone. Fair enough. But here's the most important question: How will you deal with the challenges you face? Are you going to get rid of your kitchen? Stop shopping at the supermarket? Resolve never to celebrate the holidays? Bar guests at the door? Of course not. Besides, your kitchen, the supermarket, the holidays, and guests aren't really the problem. Rather, the problem is the habits you've developed in response to these aspects of your food environment.

My solution: *change your habits.* Take control of the situation, bust your old habits, and learn new, better, more creative habits.

Here's how.

Consider the following scenes in your home. Check the habits that apply to your behavior; then use these *habit busters* to help you avoid Unstructured Eating.

Home Layout: "Food Areas" and "Nonfood Areas"

You keep your home heavily stocked with food ( ). Some of the foods available there are your favorite "problem foods," ( ) and you tend to dip into them frequently ( ). In addition to regular foods for family use, you also stock special items for guests and for your own sudden cravings ( ). You store foods not only in the kitchen but also in the living room ( ), bedroom ( ), and the room where you watch TV ( ), where it's easy to do mindless munching ( ).

Habit Busters:

- Store foods only in the kitchen, not in any other rooms.
- Eliminate snack foods, especially your behavioral "problem foods," from routine storage.
- Throw out party foods you've saved "just in case" for unexpected guests.
- Teach your kids not to leave their snacks lying around to tempt you.
- Keep foods out of the living room, the TV room, and other areas that you designate as nutritional "no-fly zones."

If you can avoid making your home into a nutritional minefield, you're far less likely to trigger the bombs!

Menu Planning

You generally give little thought to what you eat ( ). In fact, you often decide what to buy at the last moment ( ). You think of others first and yourself last so that you prepare what they want and not what you need ( ). The only time you think ahead is when you have a craving ( ). You often have no idea what you'll eat except just before a meal ( ).

Habit Busters:

- Buy a cookbook with healthy recipes (with nutrition analyses) to help you plan.
- Structure each week's meals a week in advance—perhaps at a designated time, such as Sunday night.
- Note your planned meals in the Structure House Diary each week.
- Use your food group and calorie guides to plan meals.

Remember: Structuring your meals is your best defense against problematic eating habits.

Making a Shopping List

You don't prepare a shopping list ( ), since you aren't really sure what you'll be eating anyway ( ). Or you make a list with just a few items you *think* you may need ( ). All of your lists are based on whim and impulse rather than on planning ( ). You figure you'll just go to the store, follow your hunches, and hope for the best ( ).

Habit Busters:
- Plan your meals first, then determine the ingredients you need to buy.
- Using your menu plan, figure out the quantities of items to purchase—how many pounds of meat or vegetables, how many packages of prepared items, etc.
- Group the foods according to your supermarket layout to facilitate shopping and avoid "trolling" for unneeded treats and problem foods.
- Make sure you have the ingredients you need for each recipe in the menu plan, which will avoid improvising with more problematic ingredients or going off your plan.
- Avoid purchasing foods that aren't on the list.

Too much planning? Not at all! If you think ahead, you'll save yourself time and effort later. Why? Because your efforts will short-circuit Unstructured Eating by eliminating problem foods before they ever come into the house.

Shopping

When you go shopping, you generally haven't eaten for a while, so you arrive at the store hungry ( ). Since you aren't sure what you're going to fix for your meals, you tend to buy items you hadn't planned to purchase ( ). You also do "impulse buying" in response to the store's displays ( ), free samples ( ), in-store announcements ( ), and other marketing tactics ( ). You end up leaving with all kinds of foods you hadn't expected to purchase ( ).

Habit Busters:
- Schedule shopping trips after you've eaten one of your regular Structured meals.
- Shop only from a prepared list.
- See your task as time-limited and goal-oriented: just get the items on your list and clear out.
- Avoid interior aisles, which often have less crucial, more tempting foods.
- If possible, delegate shopping to other family members, or consider using only shopping and delivery services.

The less time you spend hunting and gathering, the more likely you'll stay Structured.

Storing Food

On arriving home from the supermarket, you leave some goodies out on the kitchen table or on the counters ( ). You fill the refrigerator and the kitchen cabinets with foods in easy-access packages ( ). Many of the containers have see-through wrappers ( ) or enticing pictures ( ) of the food inside. Every time you open the fridge, the sight of all those tasty items drives you crazy ( ).

Habit Busters:
- Store foods in non-see-through containers (such as opaque plastic bowls or disposable aluminum pans); cover with aluminum foil instead of plastic wrap so that you can't see the contents. Label with stickers so you know what's inside without opening the containers and feeling tempted.
- Store food in individual-serving-size containers so that your meals are portion controlled. You can store the leftovers in the freezer or refrigerator and then take out the exact serving that you need, which will help you avoid overeating.
- Store only foods that need to be cooked before eating, which presents one more step to take before Unstructured Eating.
- Store all foods in the fridge or in cabinets, not on countertops, open shelves, or tables.

Out of sight, out of mind? Maybe, maybe not. But even a little forethought will save you a world of trouble by storing food in ways that aren't so tempting.

Food Preparation

When it's time to prepare a meal, you open up the cabinets and refrigerator and grab whatever is handy ( ). You nibble and taste the food as you work ( ). Because you haven't planned your meal, you feel rushed ( ), which adds to your stress and tempts you to eat to ease your tension ( ). Perhaps the members of your household like different foods, so you have to prepare several different meals ( ), and so you taste each of many dishes as you cook ( ).

Habit Busters:

- Prepare only one meal for the entire family.
- If you must prepare several meals, fix simple ones, since complex recipes will guarantee more time spent in the kitchen.

'Tis the gift to be simple. By limiting the number of separate dishes you fix and using straightforward recipes, you'll avoid many habits that come from more elaborate efforts.

Serving the Meal

When the time comes to serve the meal, you put all the items in bowls and place them on the table ( ). This situation prompts you to serve each member of the family, and it's easy to sample some of the dishes repeatedly as you proceed ( ). You finally sit down, exhausted and stressed, and you put a lot of food on your plate ( ) because you feel you deserve a reward after all this work.

Habit Busters:

- Plan appropriate portions of food for each member of your family.
- Fill the plates at the kitchen counter, then carry the plates to the table to avoid having serving dishes full of food at the table, which tempts you to have seconds and thirds.
- Focus on the visual appeal and taste combinations of food rather than just the quantity on your plate.
- If possible, avoid using large plates, which may dwarf portions of food and make them look inadequate.

Enjoy your meal as a family. By all means give teens the portions their growing bodies need. But avoid using the serve-at-the-table or buffet approach that so easily leads to habitual overeating.

Eating the Meal

You start eating rapidly ( ). You don't chew your food adequately ( ), you don't put down your utensils between mouthfuls ( ), and you finish hastily ( ). You see that food is still in the bowls in front of you, so you take seconds ( ), which upsets you but doesn't stop you from doing it ( ). You eat too much but don't really pay attention to what you eat ( ).

Habit Busters:
- Wait a moment before eating to savor the aromas, delight in the appearance, and anticipate the pleasure of your meal.
- Set down utensils between mouthfuls to avoid rushing and "scarfing" your meal.
- Truly taste and enjoy what you're eating—focus on quality, not just quantity.
- Slow down so that your meal will last at least twenty minutes.
- Eat while seated rather than "on the go"—while doing household chores, talking on the phone, or multitasking in other ways.
- Don't eat while watching TV, reading, or using the computer; just enjoy your meal!
- Enjoy the meal as family time, not just as a nutritional pit stop.

It's amazing how many people are oblivious to the food they eat! Eating has not just become habitual, it's almost robotic. My recommendation: Be mindful of what you eat. Focus on being fully aware of the aromas, tastes, and textures as you savor each bite. If you can truly experience your meal rather than cruise through it on autopilot, you'll feel much more satisfied and less tempted to overeat. (I'll have much more to say about the subject of Mindful Eating in Chapter 10.)

Cleaning Up

When everyone leaves the table, you're stuck with cleaning up on your own ( ). There are a lot of leftovers ( ), so, while emptying the pots and putting food away, you find yourself nibbling once again ( ). You're really exhausted by now, which prompts you to eat as a "payback" for your fatigue ( ).

Habit Busters:

- Clean up right after eating rather than leaving food out longer, which will tempt you to go back for more.
- Delegate cleanup tasks, or else have family members work as a team, which speeds up the process.
- After the meal, sprinkle pepper on any food that remains on individual plates to make it unappetizing.
- Don't leave any extra servings of food in pans or on the table; pack them up and refrigerate them if they're usable or throw them out if they're not.

Okay, so cleanup is a chore. Everyone hates it, and it's a risky time because of the hazards it presents for more Unstructured Eating. But it's also an opportunity to stay Structured and to avoid setting yourself up for trouble later in the day—or tomorrow.

Entertainment and Holidays

Your parties, holiday celebrations, and family occasions focus on food as the main event ( ). You prepare huge quantities of food as the chief expression of your hospitality ( ). Holiday and party foods are invariably fat-intensive ( ), sugar-laden ( ), or both. Overeating at such times isn't just accepted in your household, it's expected and encouraged ( ).

Habit Busters:

- All holiday meals require planning, so why not make Structure part of your plan? Recipes that are both healthy and delightful are now readily available for every kind of special occasion.
- Although eating is a wonderful part of every celebration, food doesn't have to be the whole focus of what you do with your guests. Make sure you plan enjoyable activities *other* than eating.

For parties, many healthy alternatives to standard fare exist. Salsa and low-calorie dips (210 calories and 300 calories per jar, respectively) are a great replacement for regular creamy dips (800 to 1,000 calories per jar). Carrots, plum tomatoes, and other veggies—or even baked tortilla chips—are far healthier to dip than potato chips and fried tortilla chips.

Set Priorities

Maybe you don't have trouble with all these habits. Perhaps you feel more tempted to eat while shopping and less so while preparing meals, or perhaps it's the other way around. Or perhaps you struggle with several of these issues simultaneously. Everyone's different.

My recommendation: Review the items you checked and note the *three* habits that you find most problematic. Prioritize them as Habits 1, 2, and 3 according to the level of challenge they present to you. These priorities will set your agenda. Then write down which of the Habit Busters you'll use to deal with each particular food habit. Your agenda will give you specific tasks to practice.

Why set priorities at all? Let's face it: It's difficult to change lots of habits at once. It's easier and more effective to focus on three (at most) at a time. Even then, it's best to tackle them one at a time. Doing so will let you focus on a manageable set of issues. Make some changes, grow comfortable with them, and master new skills before moving on. You might focus on compiling better lists for grocery shopping, for instance, before you tackle the issues you face in the supermarket itself. Give yourself time to experiment. Look at the process as a puzzle or a game, not as a chore. Allow time to try out options and see what really works for you. Go ahead, try it. Replacing even one old, problematic habit with a new, productive one will give you great satisfaction and boost your confidence. Then you can move on to change another habit—and another, and another. Comfortable, incremental change is the most effective approach for achieving long-term success.

Put Your Commitment into Writing

Now make a commitment to change. Suppose that your most problematic habit is Unstructured Eating when guests show up unannounced. You want to be hospitable, so you habitually serve cake, cookies, and other rich, high-calorie foods. But having these items in the house is a big problem. It's better not to have them around at all! But then how are you going to deal with entertaining in the future? Are you going to stop inviting friends over? Of course not—that's out of the question. A better approach: Plan to have healthy foods available from the start. Write down your commitment: "In my newly structured kitchen, I'll stock delicious, healthy foods." Then follow through on your commitment. Offer noncaloric or low-cal beverages and some fresh fruit salad. Serve veggies and low-cal dip. You have all kinds of options to choose from.

Will your written "vow" settle the issue? I hope so. In any case, writing down your commitment to change will strengthen your resolve.

Some examples:

- "On Sunday evenings, I'm going to plan the next week's dinners."
- "I'm going to make sure I've always eaten lunch before I go shopping at the supermarket."
- "From now on, I'm going to focus on really enjoying each meal rather than using mealtimes to watch TV, read the paper, or pay bills."
- "I'll use simpler recipes now rather than feeling obliged to make fancy meals that take longer and tempt me to nibble."
- "From now on, I'll clean up quickly to get the food out of sight and out of mind— and everyone else in the family will pitch in, too."

Let's face it: you can't change all your habits at once. But changing just two or three at a time can be done. Use your imagination. Make a commitment—and make a plan. Change won't happen overnight, and that's okay. Be persistent. Take the long view. Even after only a week or two of changing your habits, you'll feel great about the progress you've made.

TASK 2: PLAN YOUR MENUS

The most important step you can take toward Structured Eating is menu planning. By using the Structure House Diary, you can structure each day ahead of time, then plan meals accordingly. Here's how.

Control Calories and Portions

To lose weight safely, you need to determine the minimum number of calories that's healthy for you to consume each day and still lose weight. This number will be based on your estimated metabolic rate and activity level. Knowing that figure shouldn't be guesswork; fortunately, there's a straightforward formula you can use to find out the answer. See Appendix 2 for the Mifflin–St. Jeor equation. A nutritionist or dietician can also make the calculation for you.

Either way, you now have an accurate, nutritionally sound figure to use as you start planning your menus, your caloric intake, and your weight loss program.

This level should allow you enough calories that you don't feel deprived and dissatisfied. There's no law that says you must eat the minimum number of calories that is healthy for you until you get to your goal weight! In fact, you may find that over time, you may need to *increase* your calories in a healthy, structured manner to help you stick with your weight loss plan. It's better to lose weight at a slower rate than to give up and resume overeating.

Determining calories and controlling portions are a crucial part of the Structure House program. It's all too easy to gain weight simply eating a *little* too much food—even if it's healthy food—each day. An extra 100 calories of healthy food each day accounts for 10 pounds of body fat a year, or 100 pounds a decade. It's easy to let this food "slip under the radar"; research shows that most people underestimate the amount they eat. The most foolproof method for controlling calories and portions is to weigh and measure your foods—at least until you begin to recognize portion sizes.

Understand the Food Groups

Each day, you need to consume an appropriate balance of protein, carbohydrates, and fat, as well as a variety of vitamins, minerals, and other beneficial nutrients. But you don't need to calculate the grams of saturated fat or milligrams of cholesterol each day in order to eat a heart-healthy diet. Nor do you need to calculate the amount of fiber or each of the vitamins and minerals you need each day.

The simplest method of obtaining the right balance of nutrients is to visualize a healthy plate. When you are eating a healthy diet, half of your lunch or dinner plate will be vegetables, a quarter will be animal protein, and a quarter will be starch. You can have a serving of fruit and dairy on the side.

However, our favorite menu-planning guide at Structure House is the American Diabetes Association's exchange lists.[1] We regard the ADA exchange lists as the best guide for getting the right number of calories of a balanced variety of healthy foods. These lists are immensely valuable not just for diabetics but for anyone concerned with good nutrition. The ADA exchange lists are readily available from nutritionists, dieticians, and the American Diabetes Association itself. (Visit their Web site at: www .diabetes.org.) See also Appendix 3.

Note, however, that servings within each food group will have approximately the same number of calories only if you use the correct portion listed. (An "exchange" is essentially the same thing as a portion.) For example, a serving from the starch group has 80 calories. Servings are small—only ⅓ of a cup of rice or pasta or a 1-ounce slice of bread. (A typical restaurant serving of pasta, on the other hand, is 3 cups, or 700 calories before adding the sauce.)

How can you most effectively plan your meals using the exchange lists as a guide? Of course, one approach would be to consult a nutritionist or dietician for advice—an easy way to map out a nutritional strategy. Alternatively, you can easily obtain the American Diabetes Association's exchange list materials through this organization's Web site and do your own planning. The key is to plan meals based on the number and kind of exchanges (portions) suitable for the calorie level you intend to consume.

The following table can give you an overview of the portions available at various levels. (Keep in mind that portions are quite small—definitely *not* equivalent to restaurant-sized portions!)

Table 5.1 Number of Exchanges (Portions) for Each Calorie Level

Type of Food	Number of Calories					
	1,000	1,200	1,500	1,800	2,000	2,500
Starches and Breads	4–5	5–6	7	8	9	11
Fruits	2	3	3	4	4	6
Milk and milk products	2	2	2	3	3	3
Vegetables	3+	3+	4+	4+	5+	5+
Meat and meat alternatives	5	5	6	6	6	8
Fats*	1.5	3	4	4	5	6

* Source: American Diabetes Association. Used with permission.

Now let's take a quick tour through the food groups to see how each contributes to good nutrition and Structured Eating.

The Starches and Breads Group

Contrary to what some popular diet books suggest, carbohydrates in foods like starches are *not* the only major culprit in weight gain. You can gain weight by eating more than the maintenance level of calories of *any* type of food, even protein. But the most likely culprit in weight gain is probably fat. Nutrient-rich starches are, in fact, definitely part of any well-balanced weight loss plan. Within this food group, make sure you have at least three servings of a whole-grain food each day. At least half of the grain products you consume each day needs to be whole grain. Otherwise it's difficult to get enough fiber, some of the trace minerals, and B vitamins.

Note, however, that selecting whole-grain bread can be tricky. Many wheat, multigrain, oat bran, rye, and pumpernickel breads aren't actually 100 percent whole grain. In the next chapter of this book, "Be Structured at the Supermarket," you'll learn how to pick a whole-grain bread. This group includes high-water-soluble-fiber foods such as oatmeal, dried beans, and legumes, which appear to lower LDL cholesterol as well as help regulate blood glucose levels after meals.

The Fruits and Vegetables Groups

These two groups abound in hundreds of plant nutrients, many of which are only now being identified. These plant nutrients are thought to prevent or slow the growth of cancer, as well as protecting your heart, vision, and genes.

Plant nutrients are responsible for the variety of beautiful colors in the foods in the fruit and vegetable groups. To get the variety of plant nutrients you need to protect against disease, eat as many colors (green, red-orange, red-purple, and blue-purple) of fruits and vegetables as you can each day. In particular, emphasize the deep green and orange vegetables. You may be daunted by the number of servings recommended from the fruit and vegetable groups each day. But a serving isn't as large as you may imagine. A serving of a fruit or vegetable is only about one cup raw or about ¾ cup cooked. The food exchange lists give you more exact servings for the purpose of calorie counting.

The Milk and Milk Products Group

When you lose weight, you're not only losing body fat—you may be losing bone mass as well. For this reason, make sure you get enough calcium.

Current recommendations are for three servings of low-fat dairy products each day to meet your calcium requirement. One serving is 1 cup of low-fat or nonfat milk, or else calcium-fortified soy milk or 6 ounces of low-fat or nonfat yogurt. Many Americans, particularly those who are dieting, don't get the recommended amount of dairy products. If you find it difficult to get three cups of nonfat or lowfat dairy products each day, you'll need to take a calcium supplement. Calcium is absorbed just as well from a well-chosen calcium supplement as it is from a dairy product, particularly if (as in the case of calcium carbonate supplements) you take it with meals.

The Meat and Meat Alternatives Group

Dietary saturated fat (and, to a lesser extent, cholesterol) raise the detrimental low-density-lipoprotein levels in our blood more than any other component of food. Unfortunately, much of the saturated fat and cholesterol we eat is actually hidden in foods, particularly in foods in the meat and meat alternatives group. A 3-ounce serving of cheese has about the same amount of saturated fat as 6 teaspoons of butter. In fact, cheese is the only member of the highest-fat meat and meat alternatives category in the exchange lists. For this reason, most of your selections from this group each day should come from the lean and very lean categories. These lower-saturated-fat categories include fish, shellfish, chicken, and turkey (white meat without the skin); lean beef (round, flank, sirloin); cheese that has no more than 3 grams of fat per ounce; and cottage cheese that is no more than 4 percent fat.

An easy way to limit your intake of saturated fat and cholesterol is to have only 6 ounces (or serving equivalents) from this group each day (preferably from the lean and very lean categories), or else make sure that no more than one fourth of your plate is from this group. (Be careful about the size plate you use. At Structure House, we use a luncheon-sized plate as a dinner plate.) Some of the selections from the meat and meat alternatives group (egg whites, tofu, fat-free cheese, and soy meat alternatives) have virtually no saturated fat and cholesterol, so they don't need to be limited as long as you aren't exceeding your total calories for the day.

For cardiac health, it's recommended that most people limit their consumption of egg yolks to 4 per week. If you have heart disease, diabetes, or many risk factors for heart disease, a limit of 2 yolks per week may be more ideal.

The American Heart Association now recommends that all Americans have at least two meals of fish per week (preferably fatty, cold-water fish) in order to get adequate amounts of the beneficial omega-3 fatty acids that protect our hearts. So if you'd sometimes like to exceed the suggested limit of fish, poultry, and lean meat each day, do so with fish. Omega-3 fatty acids are also present in small amounts in some plant foods (canola, soybean, walnut oil). (Note, however, that your body utilizes the omega-3 fatty acids in fish better than the omega-3 fatty acids in plant foods.)[2]

The Fats Group

The *type* of fat you eat influences your risk of heart disease more than the *amount* you eat. To protect against heart disease, keep your saturated fat intake at *less than 10 percent* of your total calories. People who are at higher risk of heart disease need to keep their saturated fat intake at *less than 7 percent* of total calories. To achieve these goals, you need to eat more of the healthy monounsaturated fats (olive, canola, and peanut oils, nuts, and peanut butter) and polyunsaturated fats (corn, safflower, and soybean oils, soft margarines, and mayonnaise) and restrict your intake of the saturated fats in foods such as butter, bacon, cream, and sour cream. (Nuts may be a behavioral problem food for some people. You may need to decide if you will be able to regulate the amount of nuts or peanut butter you eat if you have a supply in your house.) You must also limit the amount of saturated trans–fatty acids that you eat. Many of the trans–fatty acids in the American diet come from processed foods that contain hydrogenated oils (hard margarines, snack foods) and deep-fried restaurant foods.

Some further suggestions[3]:

- Limit meat, fish, poultry, and cheese to 6 ounces a day. Include meat alternatives to reach 8 servings from the Meat and Meat Alternatives group on 2,500 calories.
- Allow up to 4 egg yolks per week if your cholesterol levels are normal.
- Choose added fats that are mono- and polysaturated.

If your LDL level is over 100 mg/dL, you should have no more than 200 milligrams of cholesterol and no more than 7 percent of calories from saturated fat. You can achieve this by:

- Limiting meat, fish, poultry, and cheese to 5 ounces a day.
- Allowing 2 egg yolks per week.
- Choosing added fats that are mono- and polyunsaturated.

However, if you wish to control your weight, you must also be attentive to the amount of fat you eat. Make sure that the amount of healthy fat you eat fits into your total calorie goal for the day.

Don't Ignore Healthy Foods Just Because of Their Calories!

Sometimes people avoid great sources of nutrition just because their caloric values seem too scary. This is a big mistake. Some of these foods are crucial sources of important nutrients. And some calorie-dense foods are actually more satisfying, so you're less likely to overeat than if you focus only on "low-calorie" foods. Some recommendations:

- Choose high-calorie items from the fruits and vegetables groups. Choose grapes, bananas, or raisins instead of strawberries and melons. Choose peas, corn, potatoes, or sweet potatoes instead of lettuce wedges.

- Increase servings of mono- and polyunsaturated fats such as olive or canola oil, margarine, etc.

- Include healthy caloric liquids (such as milk and orange juice) with your meals. They can help you get enough calcium and vitamin C and enough calories without having to eat so much food.

- Use regular products rather than diet products. For example, use regular 100 percent whole-wheat bread rather than diet bread.

- Choose fruits that are higher in calories for their volume. In addition to having low-calorie vegetables from the vegetables group, choose some of the higher-calorie starchy vegetables from the starches group.

- Increase servings of healthy mono- and polyunsaturated fats. Rather than having diet dressing from a bottle, make vinaigrette with olive oil and balsamic vinegar. Also, sauté your vegetables in a little olive oil and garlic. Research suggests that dieters eat more vegetables when they are "dressed up" rather than simply steamed. They also control their weight better.

Get the Most Nutrients for Your Calories

To get the most bang for your buck, nutritionally speaking, you need to emphasize vegetables, fruits, whole grains, and lean sources of protein while limiting fat (particularly solid fat), sugar, and alcohol. Many of the foods that have the most nutrients for the calories are also low-calorie-dense foods, which means that they provide a lot of volume for the number of calories. (See the box on page 100 for a comparison of the energy densities of a wide range of foods.)

Structure House participants are often surprised to discover how much food they can eat and still lose weight. Some even find that it isn't always easy to finish their meals. Healthy diets that are high in fiber and

Energy Density of Foods
(Calories per Gram)

Very Low Energy Dense

Lettuce	0.1
Strawberries	0.2
Tomatoes	0.2
Broccoli	0.3
Vegetarian vegetable soup	0.3
Milk, skim	0.4
Chicken, rice, vegetable soup	0.5
Oranges	0.5

Low Energy Dense

Oatmeal, prepared with water	0.6
Yogurt, fat-free, plain	0.6
Tofu	0.6
Grapes	0.7
Orange roughy, broiled	0.9
Bananas	0.9
Potato, baked with skin	1.1
Tuna, canned in water	1.1
Rice, white, long-grain, cooked	1.3

Medium Energy Dense

Chicken breast, roasted, no skin	1.7
Bread, whole wheat	2.5
Potato chips, fat-free	2.7
Ground beef, lean, broiled	2.7
Raisins	3.0
Snackwells Cookie Cakes Devil's Food Fat Free	3.0
French fries	3.2
Pizza Hut pan pizza with pepperoni	3.3
Dunkin' Donuts glazed donut	3.5
PowerBar Performance bar	3.5
Swiss cheese	3.8
Hard pretzels	3.8
Popcorn, air-popped, plain	3.8
Slim-Fast Diet Bar	3.9

Very High Energy Dense

Burger King onion rings	4.0
Granola bar, oats and honey	4.3
Granola bar, chewy chocolate chip	4.3
Quaker 100% Natural Granola without milk	4.6
Brownie	4.7
Bacon	5.0
Milk chocolate bar	5.4
Cheese puffs	5.4
Peanuts, roasted	5.9
Potato chips	6.5
Butter	7.2
Oil, vegetable	8.8

moderate in fat provide much more volume for the number of calories than the typical American diet.

Emphasize Diversity

Particularly within the lower-calorie-dense food groups (vegetables, fruits, and nonfat and low-fat milk and yogurt), research has found that people who eat the greatest variety of vegetables have a *lower* percentage of body fat than those who eat the least. People who eat the greatest variety of higher-calorie foods tend to have a *higher* percentage of body fat than those who eat the least. Nevertheless, the greater variety you eat, the more likely it is that you'll get all of the nutrients you need. Allow yourself enough variety that you feel satisfied with your food plan and can stick with it.

Control Sodium Intake

You may not know it, but sodium is present is almost every food you eat. Animal foods are generally lower in sodium than processed foods, but they're higher in sodium than plant foods. Although processed foods often have a high sodium content, fresh, unprocessed foods contain sodium, too. Even fresh fruits and vegetables have small amounts of sodium. Restaurant foods and processed foods generally have the highest levels of all.

Why are these facts important? Because they have a big impact on your health. To maintain a healthy blood pressure—and to control elevated blood pressure if you're already hypertensive—you should consume no more than 2,300 milligrams of sodium a day—and, ideally, 1,500 milligrams. Keep in mind that one teaspoon of salt has about 2,300 milligrams of sodium. This *doesn't* mean that you can add one teaspoon of salt to your foods each day! Because of how powerfully sodium affects your blood chemistry and, as a result, your blood pressure, this is a crucial issue for your long-term health.

How can you avoid consuming excess sodium? The easiest way is by remembering that nature provides you with the right amounts in whole, unprocessed foods. You don't need to count the amount of sodium in every food you eat—that's just too much work. A better approach is simple: Don't add salt when you cook, don't add salt at the table, and limit your intake of higher-sodium processed foods and restaurant foods. Examples of higher-sodium processed foods include canned goods and other items that have a long shelf life. And remember: some condiments such as soy sauce, salsa, and ketchup also add sodium to your diet.

TASK 3: PREPLAN WHENEVER POSSIBLE

Preplanning your meals saves you time and effort in the long run, saves you the trouble of making extra trips to the supermarket, and helps to make healthy eating a priority. The result: Structured Eating is easier when you plan your meals than when you wing it. Deciding what to eat at the last minute is a recipe for Unstructured Eating.

Day by Day . . . or Even a Week at a Time

What does Structured Eating look like in black and white? There's an almost infinite variety of ways that you can plan nutritious, healthy, delightful meals and stay Structured. Planning meals may sound like work, but in fact looking ahead a day, a week, or even several weeks at a time will save you lots of effort in the long run. Here's what a week's worth of meal-by-meal menus—selected almost at random from our dieticians' database—looks like at Structure House:

MONDAY BREAKFAST	calories	MONDAY LUNCH	calories	MONDAY DINNER	calories
raisin bran	140	1 turkey vegetable wrap	250	5 oz fish Parmesan	220
1 c skim milk	90	1 c butternut squash soup	70	⅔ c lemon thyme rice	170
1 slice whole wheat toast	90	1 c grapes	110	1 c green beans	30
1 tsp margarine*	30			½ c blueberries	110
total	350	total	430	total	465

* Structure House serves trans-fat-free margarine.

TUESDAY BREAKFAST

	calories
2 strawberry and cheese blintzes	143
1 c melon	50
½ c yogurt	50
total	**243**

TUESDAY LUNCH

	calories
2 vegetable frittata	220
1 c gazpacho	76
½ pita	85
2 oz carrot sticks	20
total	**401**

TUESDAY DINNER

	calories
grilled marinated flask steak	310
6 oz sweet potato	160
½ c yogurt	50
1c strawberries	50
total	**570**

WEDNESDAY BREAKFAST

	calories
3-egg mushroom-and-onion omelet	55
1 whole wheat bagel	120
½ c pineapple	40
¼ c cottage cheese	45
total	**260**

WEDNESDAY LUNCH

	calories
salad with grilled chicken and blue cheese	238
1 pita	170
banana	90
total	**498**

WEDNESDAY DINNER

	calories
beef-stuffed pepper	230
1 baked potato	160
½ c snap peas	25
1 tsp margarine	30
total	**445**

THURSDAY BREAKFAST

	calories
⅔ c scrambled eggs	90
1 English muffin	130
½ c mandarin oranges	35
½ c yogurt	50
total	**305**

THURSDAY LUNCH

	calories
southwestern black bean turkey salad w/ cilantro and lime dressing	323
1 c yogurt	100
1 c pears	60
total	**483**

THURSDAY DINNER

	calories
4 oz chicken with spinach and mushrooms	255
1 c lemon walnut broccoli	90
⅓ c herb couscous	80
½ c blueberries	45
total	**470**

FRIDAY BREAKFAST

	calories
4-egg-white omelet w/ vegetables	70
2 slices whole wheat toast	180
1 c strawberries	50
total	**300**

FRIDAY LUNCH

	calories
Philly cheesesteak—stuffed baked potato	315
1 c coleslaw	80
1 apple	80
6 oz vegetable soup	40
total	**515**

FRIDAY DINNER

	calories
5 oz tomato caper fish	215
⅔ c brown rice	140
1 c steamed zucchini	30
½ c pineapple	40
total	**425**

SATURDAY BREAKFAST

	calories
Cheerios	60
1 c skim milk	90
1 banana	90
2 egg whites	30
total	**270**

SATURDAY LUNCH

	calories
⅓ c turkey salad	145
2 slices whole wheat toast	180
1 slice lettuce/tomato	7
½ c grapes	55
½ c bean chowder	75
total	**462**

SATURDAY DINNER

	calories
4 oz filet mignon	240
1 oz mustard sauce	20
½ c roasted onions and peppers	48
2 c spinach salad	10
dressing	40
⅓ c pecan brown rice	88
½ c applesauce	50
total	**496**

SUNDAY BREAKFAST		SUNDAY LUNCH		SUNDAY DINNER	
	calories		calories		calories
spicy Mexican omelet	125	½ hummus sandwich	162	sweet and sour chicken	256
2 oz salsa	16	1 c turkey rice soup	140	⅓ c brown rice	70
2 oz sour cream topper	40	2 broccoli spears	20	1 c strawberries	50
1 whole wheat bagel	120	1 c peaches	60	½ c yogurt	50
1 c tropical fruit	90	½ c yogurt	50	**total**	**426**
total	**391**	**total**	**432**		

You can preplan menus that suit your own tastes, culinary skills, and budget. For the specifics of how we cook tasty meals at Structure House, see Appendix 3, The Structure House Menu Sampler.

The Joy of Quick and Easy Cooking

Simple recipes are far less likely to result in high-calorie meals. Elaborate, time-consuming recipes usually mean higher-calorie meals—and they give you more time and opportunity to nibble as you cook. Some studies suggest that people who eat relatively simple meals tend to be leaner. In addition, consumption of a greater variety in most food groups (combination foods, snack foods, meat/protein foods, and starchy foods) is associated with a higher percentage of body fat. My recommendation: Cook simply and eat simply.

Here's how:

Buy Preprepped Items

Buying preprepped ingredients (or prepping them yourself ahead of time) will save you time, which will encourage you to plan your meals and stay Structured. Preprepped foods you can purchase at most supermarkets include:

- Fresh produce (prewashed salad greens, peeled carrots, peeled and/or chopped garlic, broccoli slaw, vegetable mix for stir-fry, cherry tomatoes, diced or cubed fruit)
- Dairy goods (grated cheese, sliced cheese, cubed cheese, egg whites in cartons)
- Meat (cubed beef, ground turkey breast, boneless/skinless chicken)

- Canned fruits in water or juice
- Frozen fruits and vegetables (avoid those packed in sauces and syrups)

You can also preprep foods yourself by cutting or chopping produce, meat, or cheese ahead of time and storing in appropriate portions for later use.

Prepare and Freeze Meals for Later Use

Freezing batches of food you've prepared can be a wonderful time saver. You can cook meals ahead of time—including quiches, soups, lasagnas, and eggplant parmesan—then freeze portions to use on a night when you're too busy to cook.

Here are some tips for stocking your freezer:

- Cool foods (preferably in the refrigerator) before freezing. Foods that have been cooled before freezing will freeze more rapidly, and rapid freezing helps to retain the food's natural color, flavor, and texture.
- Freeze in portions that you'll need for one meal.
- Foods containing liquids require about a ½ inch of extra space in the container, as they will expand when frozen.
- Remove as much air as possible when packaging other foods.
- Make sure that your freezer's temperature is no higher than 0 degree Fahrenheit to maintain the quality and to extend the storage life of the food.
- User freezer-proof foils, wraps, and containers.
- Make sure that the containers' sealing edges are free of moisture and food so that they seal properly.
- Label each package or container with name, date, and portion size. Use tape, crayons, and pens that are made specifically for freezer use.
- Arrange packages so that you can use the ones that have been frozen longest before the ones that have been frozen for a shorter period of time.
- Freeze only the amount of food that will freeze within twenty-four hours (about 2 to 3 pounds of food per cubic food of storage). Overloading your freezer will slow the freezing rate, which can diminish the quality of the food.

Use Computer Software to Analyze Recipes

If you find analyzing recipes for nutritional content too difficult or time-consuming, consider this recent innovation: software programs that do it for you. They make the process easy and even fun. Among these programs are Calorie King, Dine Healthy, and Balance Log. These programs include databases ranging from three thousand to ten thousand foods. If you love computers, any one of these programs can make you a nutrition nut. They will analyze your whole diet meal by meal and provide a nutritional analysis that indicates protein, carbohydrate, fat, sodium, fiber, cholesterol, and calories. You can obtain these same data by other means, of course, but nutritional software makes the process completely painless.

Use Web-Based Resources

Another option is using Web sites that plan your menus. Here again, many options exist, but one I recommend is CaloriesCount.com. This site uses input from some of the best-respected experts in the field of obesity.

How do these sites work? Basically, they offer fee-based menu-planning data at different caloric levels. CaloriesCount.com, for instance, offers online access and support, meal plans and recipes, information on health issues and exercise, and access to expert advice through chats and feature articles. Other sites, such as WeightWatchers.com, JennyCraig .com, eDiets.com, and WebMD (www.webmd.com), all provide similar services. Although they charge a subscription fee, most of these sites offer a free trial period so that you can determine if you're interested in what they have to offer.

Structure House has no affiliation or financial relationship with any of these organizations or their Web sites.

TASK 5: OUTWIT YOUR APPETITE

Research suggests that the amount of food we eat is determined more by *the weight of the food* than by *the calories in the food*. The implication: you may tend to eat the same weight of food each day *regardless of the amount of calories the food contains*. And if you consume the same weight or volume of food but with fewer calories than usual, you will lose weight without feeling hungry.

Consider the consequences of selecting one or the other of these two foods:

Carrots   195 calories per pound
Fat-free potato chips   2,431 calories per pound

And what about picking one or the other of these two foods?

Strawberries   139 calories per pound
PowerBar Performance bar   1,600 calories per pound

Here's why these choices make so much difference. Foods that are low-calorie-dense are low in calories for the weight. These low-calorie-dense foods tend to contain a relatively high amount of water (examples: fruits, vegetables, milk, yogurt, cooked whole grains, and soups). A low-calorie-dense diet tends to be high in fiber and low in fat.

By contrast, high-calorie-dense foods tend to be dry and often high in fat (examples: nuts, chocolate bars, processed snack foods, and oils). Everyone knows that high-fat snacks like potato chips, cookies, and crackers are high in calories for their weight. You may not realize, however, that low-fat versions (such as fat-free chips and cookies) are also high in calories for their weight! Processed low-fat and fat-free foods (such as energy bars, diet bars, and pretzels) are usually higher in energy density than low-fat and fat-free foods provided by Mother Nature. Consider, for example, that cereal bars have about 4.3 calories per gram of weight, whereas apples have only 1.6 calories per gram.

Why does the weight or bulk of the food you eat have more influence over satisfying your sense of hunger than the number of calories in the food? It's because your body has many satiety (fullness) systems that send signals to the brain when you've eaten enough. Eating an adequate volume of food is necessary to activate these satiety systems.

- **Mind and eyes.** Seeing an adequate portion of appetizing food on your plate increases your expectation that you'll feel full at the end of the meal.

- **Nose and mouth.** You derive sensory pleasure from a food's aroma, "mouth feel," and taste. Since you need more time to eat a large volume of food, the taste and other sensory satiety signals transmitted to the brain last longer.

- **Stomach.** A large volume of food fills your stomach, activating stretch receptors. These stretch receptors send signals to the brain to indicate that a satisfying amount of food has been eaten. Also, as your stomach fills, it contracts rhythmically to digest the food mechanically. Your stomach contracts the same amount whether you eat a pound of high-calorie food or a pound of low-calorie food. These contractions also transmit satiety signals to the brain.

- **Liver, pancreas, small intestine, and large intestine.** As food travels through the rest of the digestive tract, your brain receives other satiety signals. For example, a large volume of food facilitates the release of cholecystokinin, "the satiety hormone," in the small intestine.

The implication: if you focus on eating low-energy-dense foods, you'll tend to feel full even though your caloric intake is relatively low. This situation outwits your appetite and clearly works to your advantages as you try to lose weight. That's what I want you to do.

In addition, the *variety* of foods you eat will make a difference. As a result of sensory-specific satiety—that is, a feeling of fullness—we tend to eat more when offered more variety. Eating a greater variety of foods from most food groups (including snacks, starches, meats, and combination foods) is associated with a higher percentage of body fat. However, eating a wide variety of foods from the vegetable group is associated with a lower percentage of body fat. Bottom line: You're better off limiting the variety of the foods you eat.

Eat Breakfast

People who eat breakfast consume diets that are lower in fat and higher in fiber, vitamins, and minerals. Statistically, people who eat breakfast tend to be leaner than those who skip this meal. Some of the evidence:

- Research by the National Weight Control Registry—a landmark study of several thousand people who have been successful at stable weight loss over an extended period of time—indicated that 78 percent of 2,959 successful weight losers ate breakfast every day of the week.[4]

- A University of Massachusetts Medical School study showed that people who skip breakfast are 4.5 times more likely to be obese than those who eat breakfast regularly.[5]

- According to research presented by the American Heart Association, people who eat breakfast are significantly (one third) less likely to be obese and diabetic than those who don't.[6]

What's this all about? Possible reasons for why breakfast is associated with leaner body weight include the possibility that eating more food in the morning may help to limit overeating later; in addition, calories eaten earlier in the day may be more satiating than the same number of calories consumed later on.

Eliminate Snacking

Studies reveal that when we aren't really hungry but we snack anyway, we don't eat fewer calories at our meals to compensate. People who snack have a higher body mass index (BMI) than those who don't.[7] Why? Many snack foods (such as pretzels, nuts, and chips) tend to be behavioral problem foods. Because we eat them by the handful, we're less likely to regulate the amount we eat of these foods. Yet intake of these foods doesn't necessarily affect our consumption of food at regular meals.

Enjoy the Delights of Water

People who drink plenty of fluid tend to be leaner. Women need at least 9 cups of fluid per day; men need at least 12. At least half of your fluid intake each day should be from water.

TASK 5: SLOW DOWN AND ENJOY COOKING

It takes time and energy to have a healthy lifestyle. Cooking at home takes more effort than eating out or grabbing take-out meals from a restaurant.

Preplanning menus takes forethought. Exercise takes time, too. None of these things happens with the wave of a magic wand.

A lot of people think of cooking as a rat race. Since life in general may *seem* like a rat race, they see time in the kitchen as just another lap around the track. Why bother?

Well, I certainly understand if you feel pressured, but I hope you can begin to see cooking in a more positive light. In times past, many cultures considered cooking—the opportunity to enjoy nature's bounty and to share it with the people you care about—as a special gift. Now we tend to regard it as a burden. A better approach: make cooking a time when you focus on the moment—the colors of the foods you're preparing, their shapes and textures, and the alchemy of transforming ingredients into a delicious meal. Healthy food is beautiful. I encourage you to make healthy meals and present them in a beautiful way, with attention to appearances. Serve your meal on attractive dishes and have flowers on the table. Make mealtime into a ritual. Do more than just eat; nurture your mind and soul as well as your body.

CHAPTER 6

Be Structured at the Supermarket: Eating Well and Losing Weight by Shopping Wisely

"I can destroy a perfect Structured day in less than five minutes of supermarket 'grazing.' Yes, destroy!!"

—Kate

Visualize your local supermarket. Now picture yourself walking in through the doorway on a routine shopping trip.

The moment you enter the store, you're in a state of sensory overload. "*Viva Italia!*" proclaim promotional posters, each showing a delectable Italian specialty. "Attention, shoppers!" declares a voice on the PA system. "Fresh-baked and piping hot, our scrumptious cinnamon buns are now available at the bakery." An employee at a display table offers you samples of a new gourmet ice cream. Aromas from the take-out section waft enticingly through the store. And all around you is food, food, food.

How can you shop sensibly in a place like that? How can you focus on buying the products you need to stay Structured? Even if you avoid indulging in the tasty samples you're offered, how can you resist loading your cart with all kinds of goodies you don't need—and never even intended to buy?

GOOD NEWS, BAD NEWS . . .

What you face in the modern American supermarket is a walk-in good-news/bad-news joke. The good news: you have a huge variety of options before you, including many healthful foods that can contribute creatively to Structured Eating. The bad news: there's an almost limitless range of not-so-healthful, heavily processed, high-calorie foods available that can damage your efforts. Shopping at the supermarket is just about the most Unstructured experience with food that you're likely to face. So be prepared for the challenge! Here are some of the trickiest areas along with a few strategies that will keep you Structured.

Shopping with Children or Grandchildren

Kids want what they want, and they want it *now*. Grocery shopping with tykes often complicates the task of Structure-oriented shopping. Before you know it, you've got a cart full of snack foods, sugary breakfast cereals, and high-calorie desserts that the kids have pleaded for. What's the solution? Ideally, you're best off shopping solo. But since that option may not be feasible, one alternative is to have the kids pick from among a narrower set of choices. Let them help decide among a few items you'd be willing to buy. Rather than asking, "What kind of cereal do you want?" pick out three acceptable products yourself, then ask, "Which one of these would you prefer?"

Navigating Hazardous Areas—the Bakery, the Deli, and the Candy Aisle

Ancient maps used to state "Here be dragons" in areas too dangerous for explorers. Some supermarket aisles are the nutritional equivalent. Why are you cruising the candy aisle, anyway? Avoid it from the start. In other areas, use your shopping list as your "map" to guide you through the store, avoid hazards, and stay on course.

Encountering "Habit Foods" or "Problem Foods"

These encounters should be expected, so don't let them sneak up on you. There you are, just minding your own business as you select some canned soups—and suddenly, out of nowhere, you see a display for buttery crackers right there in the aisle. Or you find a selection of ingredients for chocolate fondue nestled in among the berries in the produce section. Stay strong and stick with what's on your list.

Coping with Point-of-Purchase Displays, Especially of Candy

Just when you thought you were out of the woods, you face more trouble at the checkout counter! Chocolates, candy bars, and a few dozen other goodies are arrayed beside you as you wait to pay. Turn your focus toward something else. Browse a non-food-related magazine or review your shopping list. It is important to divert your gaze elsewhere. Fortunately, this problem is becoming easier to avoid these days because you can head for the no-candy aisles that many stores now maintain.

Shopping with Friends

Some people make supermarket trips a social occasion. Nice to have the company and the help, right? But this approach can backfire. Who you shop with can challenge your efforts to stay Structured. "Oh, I just love Brie!" your shopping pal exclaims. Or "I heard about this new brand of cookies that's supposed to be divine!" Not a great setup for staying Structured. Unless you have a mutual pact with your friend to avoid Unstructured Eating, run your errand on your own and plan another activity with your friend.

Dealing with Store Displays and Promotions

Walking into the store will take you through a gantlet of temptations. It takes nerves of steel to walk past all those free samples, seasonal specialties, and cooking demonstrations. The automated coupon dispensers can pique your curiosity and test your resolve. And those sales, daily specials, and two-for-one bargains: how can you resist? Well, you really can. This is a situation where your shopping list is your refuge. You're here to buy what's on the list—period. You're not visiting the store to guarantee success to the food industry's marketing campaigns. Just buy what's on the list and go home.

Despite all these distractions and temptations, you can stay Structured. Here's how to make supermarket a boost, not a burden, to Structured Eating.

BECOME A "SUPERMARKET SLEUTH"

The key to Structure-friendly shopping is to become what I call a "supermarket sleuth." This means using skills to select the products most likely to help you reach your Structured Eating goals—and avoid the products that undercut your efforts. With these skills, you'll understand individual foods more clearly and understand their nutritional benefits and drawbacks. You'll be better able to work your way through the supermarket productively.

First, though, a reminder. Structure doesn't only involve monitoring calories; it also involves learning to be aware of the nutrition available in specific foods. For this reason, shopping isn't a focus solely on calories. Here's why.

Structured Eating means that you structure your meals at home: breakfast, lunch, and dinner. You then create a shopping list that you take to the supermarket. With that list in hand, you select the items you'll be using to create your meals at home. You bring those foods home and divide up what you bought to cook the meals you've already planned. This sequence is why you don't have to fret about calories while shopping. Unfortunately, many people make the mistake of obsessing about calories while at the supermarket. You don't have to do that! Focus instead on obtaining good ingredients. Choose the *healthiest calories*, not the *fewest calories*. For example, you're better off choosing a whole-grain bread that has 70 calories a slice rather than a "light" bread that is not whole grain and has 40 calories a slice.

With these thoughts in mind, here are some skills that will help you become a supermarket sleuth and pick out good ingredients for making the meals you've planned.

Sleuthing Skill 1: Understand the Food Label— A Key to Structure

Since May 1994, the U.S. government has required a nutrition label stating "nutrition facts" on almost every food that's shipped across state lines. (Products sold at a retail site aren't obligated to post nutritional contents on a label. Your local bagel shop, for instance, doesn't need to specify a nutritional analysis because the proprietors are serving their products only to local customers.) Almost all the foods you purchase at the supermarket will have a food label on the package. What differences does it make? Look at it this way: knowledge is power—and the nutrition knowledge you gain from the food label is the power to make good choices. These choices in turn help you get Structured and stay Structured. Rather than simply buying items that *seem* appealing, you'll understand what's worth buying. This skill will be a huge advantage in your efforts to stay Structured.

The diagram on page 116 shows a sample food label.

Here are some tips on how to read and interpret the information presented in the label.

The New Label Format[1]

Sample label for macaroni and cheese

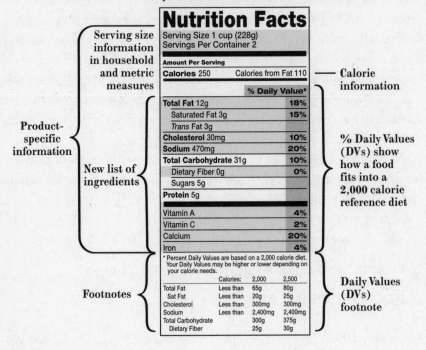

Serving size information in household and metric measures

Product-specific information

New list of ingredients

Footnotes

Calorie information

% Daily Values (DVs) show how a food fits into a 2,000 calorie reference diet

Daily Values (DVs) footnote

Nutrition Facts

Serving Size 1 cup (228g)
Servings Per Container 2

Amount Per Serving

Calories 250   Calories from Fat 110

	% Daily Value*
Total Fat 12g	**18%**
Saturated Fat 3g	**15%**
Trans Fat 3g	
Cholesterol 30mg	**10%**
Sodium 470mg	**20%**
Total Carbohydrate 31g	**10%**
Dietary Fiber 0g	**0%**
Sugars 5g	
Protein 5g	
Vitamin A	**4%**
Vitamin C	**2%**
Calcium	**20%**
Iron	**4%**

* Percent Daily Values are based on a 2,000 calorie diet. Your Daily Values may be higher or lower depending on your calorie needs.

	Calories:	2,000	2,500
Total Fat	Less than	65g	80g
Sat Fat	Less than	20g	25g
Cholesterol	Less than	300mg	300mg
Sodium	Less than	2,400mg	2,400mg
Total Carbohydrate		300g	375g
Dietary Fiber		25g	30g

Pay Attention to Serving Size

One of the most important bits of information on this label is *serving size*. Everything else on the label is meaningless unless you pay attention to this. Why? Because serving size is what gives you a context for all the other nutritional data that follows.

Here's an example of why serving size is so crucial. Some years ago, I learned that a woman in residence at Structure House at the time would habitually go through three bottles of a popular butter substitute each week—all by herself. She put gobs and gobs of this spread all over her bread, her baked potatoes, and her vegetables. She explained that her heavy use of this product couldn't possibly be a problem; after all, the label stated, "Calories: 0. Grams of fat: 0." In response to this claim, the Structure House nutritionist called up the company that manufactures this product and asked, "How many calories are in one bottle of this spread?" The answer: "Nine hundred." "And how many grams of fat in a bottle?" The answer: "Ninety." If you do the math, you'll see why this woman's use of the butter substitute was a problem. She was getting about 385 calories and 39 grams of fat simply by using that spread each day! But the manufacturer could get away with specifying "0 calories, 0 grams of fat per serving" because of technicalities in the regulations that govern use of the term "serving size" on the food label.

What's going on here? Well, many food companies make the serving sizes of their products unrealistically small. A really small serving size—such as a teaspoon of this butter substitute—results in a calorie count so low that U.S. government regulations permit the manufacturer to list the calories as zero. A low enough level of calories from fat per serving size also allows a listing of zero. But these products are *not* calorie-free! Eat enough of them, and the calories will inevitably add up. The moral of the story: you have to look at the serving size.

Make Sense of Definitions
In addition, you need to understand how manufacturers define their terms.

NUTRIENT CONTENT CLAIMS DEFINITIONS*				
	"FREE"	"LOW"	"HIGH"	"GOOD"
FAT	0.5g or less	3g or less	—	—
SATURATED FAT	0.5g or less	1g or less	—	—
CHOLESTEROL	Less than 2mg cholesterol and 2g or less saturated fat	20mg or less cholesterol and 2g or less saturated fat		
SODIUM	Less than 5mg	140mg or less	—	—
CALORIES	Less than 2 calories	40 calories or less	—	—
SUGAR	Less than 0.5mg	—	—	—
FIBER	—	—	5g or more	2.5-4.9g
OTHER NUTRIENT CONTENT CLAIMS DEFINITIONS				
"REDUCED"	25% lower in the nutrient than the comparable regular (reference) food			
"GOOD SOURCE"	Contains 10% to 19% of the Daily Value per serving			
"HIGH," "RICH IN," "EXCELLENT SOURCE OF"	Contains 20% or more of the Daily Value per serving			
"MORE," "FORTIFIED," "ADDED," "ENRICHED"	Contains at least 10% more of the Daily Value for protein, vitamins, minerals, or fiber per serving compared with the reference food			
"LIGHT," "LITE"	50% less fat than the reference food, or 50% less sodium than the reference food, food also is low calorie and low fat, or 1/3 fewer calories than the reference food, only if the reference food contains less than 50% calories from fat Light in color, Light in texture; claims must state "Light" in color or "Light" in texture			

*   Source: U.S. Department of Agriculture. These are the basic nutrient content claim definitions. Consult the Code of Federal Regulations for more details. Claims are based on Reference Amounts.

The chart on page 117 shows the definitions of nutrient content claims.[2] You need this information because it shows that some product information isn't what it seems. A "cholesterol-free food," for instance, can have up to 2 milligrams of cholesterol, since a level below 2 milligrams legally allows the company to put a zero on the label for this substance. Similarly, a "fat-free" food can have up to half a gram of fat. Look at the chart to see the specific definitions of "reduced," "lean," "high," "good source," and "light."

Put the Data to Use

Unfortunately, the food label regulations can create some ambiguous situations. On the plus side, the food label certainly makes selecting foods easier than it used to be. Serving sizes for some foods have been standardized by the USDA, which can simplify comparisons and indicate portions closer to what people normally eat. For instance, the standard "reference amount" (serving size) for margarine is 1 tablespoon; the reference amount for fresh, canned, or frozen fruit (except watermelon) is ½ cup or 140 grams; and the reference amount for cheese is 1 ounce or 30 grams. Checking the calories from fat will help you limit your fat intake—ideally, to less than 30 percent of calories from fat. Checking the data on saturated fat and cholesterol can help you make more informed choices about these factors. Checking the calories from sugar will help you limit your caloric intake of that substance, too. The same holds true of assessing your intake of sodium. If you can acquire this information, you can apply it to your advantage.

Sleuthing Skill 2: Understand Your Fat Intake

Two aspects of fat intake stand out as you do your supermarket sleuthing. One is analyzing the fat content of foods. The other is balancing your fat intake.

Analyze Fat Content

A lot of people obsess about fat. The real issue, though, is the calories from fat in a given food. This has both short- and long-term health consequences, including for cardiac health.

Calculating the percentage of calories from fat is easy. Here's what you do: look on the nutrition label, find "calories from fat," then divide that number by the total calories listed. That indicates the percentage of calories from fat. The result will be a decimal, such as .2, which would be equivalent to 20 percent.

For those of you who like formulas, here it is:

$$\frac{\text{Calories from fat}}{\text{Total calories}} = \% \text{ calories from fat}$$

I'll refer to this topic as we discuss specific foods later in this chapter.

Balance Your Fat Intake

The key issue to watch on this subject is *saturated fat*. Saturated fat is usually (but not always) from animal products—meat, cheese, butter, cream, and poultry with the skin on. It's also in tropical oils. (In fact, some of the tropical oils—palm oil, palm kernel oil, and coconut oil—are even more highly saturated than butter and lard.) Why are saturated fats a problem? It's because they raise the cholesterol level of your blood more than anything else you can possibly eat. You should also limit your intake of trans–fatty acids—oils that are saturated with hydrogen. (Trans fats are present in many snack foods, baked goods, and deep-fried restaurant foods because restaurants often cook with hydrogenated vegetable oil.) The more saturated a fat is, the more solid it will be at room temperature. For instance, butter is more saturated than stick margarine. Tub margarine is more saturated than vegetable oils. (The trans–fatty acid content of a food is now required on food labels—a development that is prompting many food companies to remove this substance from their products.)

Here are the three steps you can take to balance your intake of fats:

- First, cut your intake of saturated fats and trans fats to less than 10 percent of calories.
  - Saturated fats: meat, poultry with skin on, butter, and tropical oils
  - Trans fats: deep-fried foods, harder margarines, hydrogenated oils (in baked goods and snack foods)
- Second, use monounsaturated fats, such as canola oil and olive oil. Polyunsatu-

rated oils (such as soy, corn, safflower) and trans fat–free margarines are also healthy choices.
- Third, follow the American Heart Association guidelines for omega-3 fatty acids:
  - To decrease the risk of heart attack, eat at least two meals of fish per week (preferably lake trout, sardines, albacore tuna, or salmon).
  - If you've had a heart attack or another heart disease event, consume about 1 gram of fish oil per day.
  - If you have high triglycerides, consume 2 to 4 grams of fish oil per day *under a physician's care.*

There's a lot of confusion in the public's mind about whether butter or margarine is a healthier spread. Various contradictory news reports have spread controversy about the benefits of one product over the other. Look at Table 6.1 to see the combined trans-fat and saturated fat content of butter and margarine.

Table 6.1 Fat Content of Butter and Margarine[3]

Product (per tablespoon)	Calories	Saturated Fat (g)	Trans–Fatty Acids (g)	Combined Saturated and Trans Fatty, %
Butter	100	7	0	7
Generic margarine	100	2.5	2.5	5
Smart Balance	80	2.5	0	2.5
I Can't Believe It's Not Butter! Original	80	2	0	2
Fleischmann's original margarine	70	1.5	0	1.5
I Can't Believe It's Not Butter! Light	50	1	0	1
Brummel & Brown margarine	45	1	0	1
Take Control	45	0.5	0	0.5
Promise Fat-Free Buttery Spread	5	0	0	0

Despite the controversies over butter versus margarine, margarine basically wins regarding issues of heart health. Data in the *Journal of the American Medical Association* indicate that the use of margarine lowered LDLs in adults by 11 percent and in children by 9 percent.[4]

The overall situation is simplified by the growing number of margarines available without trans–fatty acids. Promise, Take Control, and Smart Balance are just three examples.

Sleuthing Skill 3: Understand Sodium and Additives

I'm often amazed by the number of people who worry a lot about food additives but pay little or no attention to sodium. Generally speaking, their concerns ought to be reversed.

Limit Sodium

Are you concerned about the effects of your diet on your blood pressure? I hope so—because this issue is important even if you've avoided hypertension up till now. Rates of high blood pressure increase steadily with age. Once you have high blood pressure, you run a significantly higher risk of heart disease and stroke no matter how well you control it. The best approach is to do whatever you can *not* to develop hypertension in the first place. (Optimal blood pressure is 120/80. A reading of 120–139/80–89 is considered "prehypertensive," while 140/90 or higher is regarded as indicating high blood pressure.) Once you develop high blood pressure, you have to control it. Doing so may require medication, but there are other approaches that will make a significant difference. Here are the most important means of lowering blood pressure[5]:

- **Lose excess weight.** For every twenty pounds you lose, your systolic blood pressure will go down 5 to 20 points.

- **Use the DASH diet.** This acronym stands for Dietary Approaches to Stopping Hypertension. It turns out that a low-fat diet rich in vegetables, fruits, and low-fat dairy foods works as well as blood pressure medication on mild to moderate high blood pressure.

- **Limit sodium intake.** You should consume no more than 2,400 mg of sodium per day—ideally, no more than 1,500. Doing so lowers your systolic blood pressure by 2 to 8 points. Try to limit consumption of highly processed foods and high-sodium condiments and use of the salt shaker.

- **Exercise daily.** This means 30 minutes per day of aerobic activity, such as brisk walking. The payoff: lowering your systolic blood pressure by 4 to 9 points.

- **Limit alcohol intake.** Consume no more than two drinks per day for men, one drink per day for women.

The implications? First of all, each one of these steps is important. Second, even though sodium is fourth on the list, it's extremely important to think through your consumption of this mineral and its effects on your health.

Keep Additives in Perspective

Here's the reality: every food we eat is made out of chemicals. That statement may sound shocking, but it's true. Chemicals are nature's building blocks for building everything in the universe—from galaxies to grapes, from mountains to melons. There's just no way around it. Even the purest, most perfect organic apple is made of chemicals. Even if a food item at the store lists a long string of chemicals on the nutrition label, that doesn't mean that the component parts of that food are a problem, much less that they will cause cancer. Even additives aren't necessarily the problem they seem. Many additives in food occur naturally in some other food anyway—such as calcium propionate, a preservative added to bread to prevent molding, which occurs naturally in, for example, Swiss cheese. There's more calcium propionate in an ounce of Swiss cheese than in two loaves of bread.

Despite what I'm telling you, I'm certainly concerned about additives to some degree, and your concern is legitimate. The cumulative effects of some additives remain uncertain. How should you respond to this situation? If you're concerned, I suggest that you consume foods that are as minimally processed as possible—such as by drinking real orange juice instead of processed orange drink, by fixing your own dinners rather than buying frozen diet entrees, and by using fresh ingredients rather than processed products. Better yet, eat a wide variety of foods. This strategy means that you're likely to get enough of all the nutrients you need and you won't consume too much of any one substance that could be toxic. (Are you aware that anything can be toxic in large enough amounts? There's even such a thing as water toxicity.)

Remember: if you buy fresh, unprocessed foods, you don't even have to read the labels to check for chemicals. You don't have to read the labels on fruits and vegetables, do you? You don't have to read the label on skinless chicken breast or skim milk. It's when you eat processed foods that you need to read labels.

MAKE GOOD SELECTIONS
TO HELP YOU GET STRUCTURED

All right, now you have an investigative tool kit in your possession, so let's return to the virtual supermarket we visited earlier. It's here "in the field" that you'll start to put your knowledge to use. A daunting task? Well, I think it's exciting! Your new skills in sleuthing provide you with clear vision to see which foods work to your advantage and which don't. You can't be duped anymore. Knowledge—and Structure—will put you in control.

The Meat and Poultry Department

A first consideration here is the *grade* of the meat you're buying. There are three grades of beef: *prime, choice,* and *select.* Prime and choice tend to be higher in fat; select typically has less fat. You should also consider where the cut comes from. For pork, the loin and the leg cuts are generally leaner. Loin cuts are more tender than leg cuts, though leg cuts can be tenderized by marinating or by moist-meat cooking. In poultry, white meat has less fat than dark meat. (Remember to remove the skin before eating, as poultry skin is very high in fat.)

Here are some criteria for selecting meat suitable for Structured Eating. A three-and-a-half-ounce raw portion (with the fat trimmed off) should have less than 5 grams of fat, 2 grams of saturated fat, and 95 milligrams of cholesterol. Cuts of beef that meet these criteria are eye of round, top round, veal cutlet, and lean beef of the specific brand called "Laura's Lean Beef."

Many people think of nutrition in terms of "good foods" and "bad foods." In selecting meat, there's a tendency to figure "chicken is good, red meat is bad," But nutrition is never that simple. Notice that four cuts of lean meat listed in Table 6.2 have less fat than a chicken thigh without the skin.

Table 6.2 Total Fat and Saturated Fat in Selected Meats[6]

Meat/Cut of Meat*	Grams of Saturated Fat	Grams of Total Fat
Chicken breast (without skin)	1	2
Chicken thigh (without skin)	2	7
Eye of round†	2	4
Round tip†	2	6
Top round†	1	4
Top sirloin†	2	6

* Portion size: 3 ounces cooked
† Note: All beef cuts are trimmed of fat.

These are the round and the loin cuts: eye of round, top round, round tip, top sirloin, bottom loin, top loin, and tenderloin. So these are your best bets for Structured meals.

The Deli Aisle

Now let's proceed to the deli or deli products aisle and select some lunch meats there. Which are suitable for a Structured diet, and which aren't? Sorting out your options is trickier than you may think. Here's an example: ham that the company describes as "82 percent fat-free and 18 percent fat." You'd think that only 18 percent of the product's weight comes from fat. That sounds great—but the reality is more complex than the appearance. The meat is 18 percent fat and therefore 82 percent fat-free. Remember the formula I mentioned earlier? Take the calories from fat and divide by the total calories to calculate the calories from fat. Using this method, it turns out that 75 percent of this product's calories come from fat. Is the meat company lying to you? No, it's just misleading you! What they put on the label is the *percentage of weight from fat*. What would be more informative is *percentage of calories from fat*. The best choices are lunch meats that have less than 1 gram of fat per ounce.

A Word About Meat Alternatives

Ideally, you should eat only six ounces of meat, fish, poultry, and cheese a day. Some people would prefer to have the whole six ounces at dinner, and they may feel limited by not being able to eat more than that. One response to this situation is to have a vegetarian meat alternative at lunch, which gives you the option of a larger portion of meat, fish, or poultry at dinner. Here's an overview of these meat alternatives, mostly vegetarian burgers.

One type of vegetarian burger is the original Gardenburger, made of grains and vegetables, which was the first vegetarian burger that met with commercial success. Now called "The Classic" by its manufacturer, it was the most popular vegetarian burger available for some years. It has been served at T.G.I. Friday's, the Hard Rock Cafe, the National Air and Space Museum in Washington, D.C., Disney World, many university dining halls, and Structure House. The burger contains 110 calories, 12 grams of protein, and 380 milligrams of sodium. Another brand of grain/vegetable burger is Morningstar Farms Garden Veggie Patties (100 calories, 10 grams of protein, 350 milligrams of sodium).

The second type of vegetarian burger that became popular is the soy burger, which has a taste more like meat than is true for the grain-and-vegetable burgers. Boca Burgers All American Flame Grilled Burger (90 calories, 14 grams of protein, 280 milligrams of sodium) and Morningstar Farms Classic (150 calories, 14 grams of protein, 340 milligrams of sodium) are popular brands of this type.

In addition, there are meat-extender products made from soy. They are usually rather crumbly in texture. If you make dishes with multiple ingredients, such as tacos, chili, or lasagna, you can add these soy-based meat substitutes and never notice the difference.

The Seafood Department

Proceeding to the seafood department, we find a huge array of products, many of them excellent ingredients for Structured meals. Everyone should have at least two meals of fish per week. Most fish is low in fat; however, fish with darker meat (for example, salmon) tend to have more fat than fish with white meat (examples: cod, flounder, and orange roughy). Nevertheless, you will benefit from having some of the fatty fish (mackerel, lake trout, sardines, albacore tuna, and salmon) in your diet. The reason: the omega-3 fatty acids abundant in these fish provide some protection against heart disease in several different ways. First, they help to control the rhythm of the heart. Two, they have a blood-thinning effect, which is beneficial. Three, they can lower triglycerides (a component of blood lipids). In addition, it's worth noting that omega-3 fatty acids have an anti-inflammatory effect and may be beneficial for people with rheumatoid arthritis.

The Dairy Aisle

Onward now to the dairy section! This is a crucial stop because milk and cheese are important elements in a Structured diet. They are crucial sources of calcium and vitamin D, and they can be a good source of protein as well. You need to select your dairy products carefully, however, given their issues of fat and sodium content.

Let's talk about milk first. Milk is a high-water-content food. Water is heavy, and it makes up most of the milk's weight. In whole milk, 4 percent of the weight is fat, but if you use the formula I mentioned earlier, you'll see that 51 percent of the calories are from fat. In 2 percent lowfat milk, 2 percent of the weight is fat, but 30 percent of the calories are from fat.

In 1 percent low-fat milk, 1 percent of the weight is from fat, but 22 percent of the calories are from fat. Skim milk is less than ½ percent fat by weight; less than 2 percent of the calories are from fat. A lot of people think there's hardly any difference between 1 percent milk and skim milk—but there's a *big* difference.

What are the implications for cheese? Well, cheeses are high in fat because you need lots of milk to make even a small amount of cheese. In fact, you need a gallon of whole milk to make a pound of cheese. That gallon of whole milk contains the equivalent of 32 teaspoons of butter. Depending on the brand, eight ounces of cheese contain between 800 and 880 calories and the same amount of fat as sixteen teaspoons of butter. An ounce of cheese usually has more fat than an ounce of lean red meat.

What does this mean about cheeses and their place in a Structured diet? Here are the guidelines:

- First choice: at least 50 percent reduced fat (labeled "light" or "lite")
- Second choice: at least 25 percent reduced fat (labeled "reduced fat")

The truth is that almost all cheeses are nutritionally problematic—they're too high in fat and sodium—so you should eat them only in small amounts. The least problematic cheeses are part-skim mozzarella, part-skim ricotta, and low-fat cottage. Other options include products like Cabot Creamery 50 to 75 percent reduced-fat cheeses. (Cabot Creamery has received praise for producing the best-tasting low-fat cheeses.) However, keep in mind that cheeses that are lower in fat—such as fat-free and soy cheeses—are higher in sodium.

The Bakery

Now let's move on to your supermarket's bakery or bread aisle. Many people shy away from this area altogether, but that's a big mistake. If you choose carefully, bread can be a positive part of Structured Eating.

Here's the tipoff: don't be fooled by breads with wholesome-sounding names. I'm referring to names like "earth grains," "multigrain loaf," "oat bran bread," "sprouted wheat," "honey wheatberry," "cracked wheat," "nine-grain," "twelve-grain"—the list goes on and on. Ironically, even the breads that have these natural-sounding, back-to-the-earth names often aren't 100 percent whole grain at all.

Here's why this issue is important. Kernels of grain have an external layer called the *bran*, a small area inside called the *germ*, and the rest of the internal area, which is called the *endosperm*. Eighty percent of a kernel's vitamins and minerals are in the bran and the germ. Seventy-five percent of the fiber is in the bran. So far, so good. But when you mill whole wheat flour into white flour (or brown rice into white rice), you lose most of the bran and the germ. This means that you also lose most of the vitamins, minerals, and fiber. No matter how earthy-sounding the name on the package, the bread inside is missing a lot if the manufacturer has refined so many nutrients out of it.

So how can you tell if a specific bread is really whole grain? Some guidelines:

- **These flours are *not* whole grain:** white flour, "wheat" flour, unbleached flour, enriched flour.
- **You may be surprised that even these products are *often not* whole grain:** rye bread, pumpernickel bread, diet bread, multigrain bread.

So here's a little test of your sleuthing skills. Which one of these products is 100 percent whole grain?

- **Arnold Melba Thin Rye.** Ingredients: Unbleached enriched wheat flour [flour, malted barley flour, reduced iron, niacin, thiamin mononitrate (vitamin B1), riboflavin (vitamin B2), folic acid], water, rye flour, high-fructose corn syrup, soybean oil, yeast, salt, ground caraway, sour base (lactic, acetic, fumaric acids), mono- and diglycerides, calcium propionate (preservative), datem, wheat gluten, soy lecithin, calcium carbonate.

- **Arnold Stoneground 100% Whole Wheat.** Ingredients: whole wheat flour, water, high-fructose corn syrup, wheat gluten, yeast, cracked wheat, salt, molasses, soybean oil, ethoxylated mono- and diglycerides, calcium propionate (preservative), soy lecithin.

- **La Brea Multigrain Bread.** Ingredients: unbleached flour, water, contains less than 2% of the following: dark rye flour, cracked wheat, malt powder, whole flax seeds, honey, whole millet seeds, sunflower seeds, cracked barley, salt, cracked rye, cracked triticale, yeast, graham flour, cracked millet, cracked oats, cracked corn, cracked brown rice, cracked soy beans, semolina, cracked flax seed, sour culture, niacin, reduced ion, thiamine mononitrate, riboflavin, folic acid, ferrous sulfate.

The answer: it's the middle product—Arnold Stoneground 100% Whole Wheat Bread.

Manufacturers compensate for what they've taken out by "enriching" the flour—adding thiamin, niacin, riboflavin, and iron since otherwise the values of these nutrients would be very low. Unfortunately, the companies don't enrich their products with any of the other nutrients that got lost when they milled whole grain into white flour. It's difficult to find a whole-grain product. My recommendation: size up the nutrition data carefully.

The Cereal Aisle

You may feel overwhelmed by the task of picking out a cereal that fits the Structure House program. Not to worry—here are some criteria to make the selection process easier: choose cereals with at least 5 grams of fiber and less than 8 grams of sugar per serving. Some of the cereals that meet these criteria are bran flakes, All-Bran, Shredded Wheat, Wheat Chex, and many of the Kashi brand cereals. If you don't like these options, consider mixing different types of cereals. For example, Cheerios is low in sugar, but it's also low in fiber. By contrast, Raisin Bran is high in fiber but also a little high in sugar. If you mix these two cereals together, you create a nice balance.

Don't be misled by promotions of sugary cereals for kids that claim to be "made with whole grains." If you turn the box over and check the label, you'll see that the fiber content may still be only 1 gram per serving, so the quantity of whole grains in these cereals must be fairly low.

As far as hot cereals are concerned, oatmeal is a great choice—it's a whole grain, it contains a lot of fiber, and it can even help to lower your LDL level ("bad cholesterol"). Making your own oatmeal is the best choice, as the instant varieties contain higher levels of sugar and sodium than the quick oats do. Just add some sweetener and a little fruit to create a good, hearty, healthy breakfast.

The Produce Department

We now arrive at the supermarket section that offers you one of the greatest ranges of possibilities: the produce department. The variety of fruits and vegetables available in American supermarkets has never been greater, and the quality in most parts of the country is extremely high. You can find almost any kind of produce you want. And this variety and quality are great news, because from a nutritional standpoint you almost can't go wrong.

Fruit

Here are some nutritional data typical of fresh, canned, and frozen fruit:

canned peaches in juice	55 to 80 calories per ½ cup
canned pears in juice	60 to 80 calories per ½ cup
unsweetened/natural applesauce	50 calories per ½ cup
100% apple juice	120 calories per cup
100% orange juice	120 calories per cup
100% pomegranate juice	140 to 150 calories per cup
100% grape juice	150 to 160 calories per cup

unsweetened frozen fruit:

whole strawberries	45 calorie per cup
blueberries	80 calorie per cup
peaches	60 calories per cup

A few other considerations:

- If you purchase canned fruit, buy fruit packed in its own juice; stay away from fruit packed in syrup, which adds calories without adding nutritional value.
- Frozen fruit is fine and often has nutritional content equivalent to that of fresh—as long as it doesn't contain added sugar.
- Avoid drinking more than one serving of juice a day, since drinking juice doesn't provide the fiber and other health benefits that eating fruit does.

Vegetables

One serving of just about any vegetable is 25 calories for a ½-cup cooked serving (or 1 cup raw). There are some exceptions to this rule, such as corn, peas, potatoes, butternut squash, and some others, which are higher in calories and actually belong in the starch group. Also, lettuce of various sorts and other greens have less than 25 calories per one cup raw. For maximum nutritional benefit, eat fruits and vegetables with a variety of colors, which are indicative of important nutrients.

Finally, a few suggestions:

- Frozen veggies are a great choice because they're frozen at the peak of freshness— and they don't have any added salt.
- Be careful about purchasing canned veggies because of the sodium content. (However, some companies now offer canned vegetables with no added salt.)
- Many convenient products are now available in the vegetable section: prewashed lettuce, shredded carrots, shredded cabbage, cut-up mixed veggies, carrot and celery sticks, and so forth. If you don't want to spend a lot of time in the kitchen preparing your meals, consider these options to save time.

HOMEWARD BOUND

We've completed our virtual tour of the supermarket, so it's time to visualize leaving. Your shopping cart contains the items you need—bags full of good food products that will become part of your Structured meals. What's missing? All the gimmicky and problematic products that so easily undercut and sabotage your best intentions and efforts. So now you're loading the bags into your car.

Is shopping to prepare Structured meals worth the planning it takes? Of course. Spending just a few minutes a day preparing a strategic shopping list will provide you with the "map" necessary to find your way through the tricky terrain that modern supermarkets present. Just a few sleuthing skills will provide you with the means to determine which nutritional claims are bogus and which are legitimate. Practice a little, and it'll soon be second nature.

So now you're leaving the parking lot; you're driving away. You can go home, prepare your well-planned meals, and continue your journey toward satisfying change.

CHAPTER 7

Understand the Importance of Exercise

"I also went to the gym at Structure House, and they suggested doing an hour of exercise three days a week, but I wasn't able to do it, so they said, 'Do twenty minutes a day.' But I wasn't able to do that, either. So I worked on the recumbent bike for five minutes at a time and broke it up into sessions. After the first week of my stay, I already started to feel better. There was a dramatic change in my health. I'd lost weight—maybe about 17 pounds, most of it water weight—and the loss of some weight and the exercise made me feel better physically and mentally."

—Arthur

"When I went home from Structure House, I had a game plan that I'd be able to exercise on my own, but I didn't. I eventually ended up hiring a personal trainer. She kicks my butt and keeps me honest. She makes me accountable. That's one of the most important tools I've acquired: self-accountability. Whatever you need to do to remain

self-accountable is perfectly all right. If it's hiring someone to be your personal trainer . . . that's okay."

           —Sallie

"Physically, I've always been active. But after Structure
House, I did two or three sprint triathlons and a couple of
half-marathons. I just really enjoyed my body in a completely different way."

           —Lisa

"I walk ten thousand steps a day. At lunchtime, I go to
Costco. I walk between the aisles. It's three thousand
steps. Find something that you can do. It's not such a big
deal."

           —Aaron

Exercise is a crucial component of any successful weight control program. Exercise increases your energy expenditure, since the more you
do, the more calories you burn. In addition, exercise means doing an activity other than eating. For these reasons, the Structure House program
includes a strong emphasis on exercise as a crucial component of maintaining overall good health.

 However, many overweight people are hesitant to start exercising. You
may have experienced difficulties exercising in the past that prompt concerns in the present; you may feel embarrassed to exercise because of
body image issues; or you may simply feel unsure about where to start. If
so, rest easy. Just as good health is everyone's birthright, healthful exercise,
too, belongs to everyone. Exercise needn't be a burden and can bring a
new element of enjoyment to life once you fully embrace it and make it
part of your day. The Structure House program views exercise as a "supermarket" of activities—a realm in which anyone can sample the delicacies.

 To set up and maintain the exercise program that's right for you, I urge
you to follow the five-step program described in this chapter.

STEP 1: EXPLORE EXERCISE OPTIONS

No matter what your age, gender, interests, or skill level, there is an almost limitless variety of options available to you as you explore the world of exercise.

Find Some Exercise You Can *Enjoy*

Unfortunately, many people associate exercise with work. They can't imagine doing any kind of exercise *for fun*. This is often true for people who are overweight. Yet at Structure House, I often see people's faces light up when they sample new kinds of exercise and realize that they actually enjoy them. They realize that exercise can be a kind of play—not just laborious "working out." When they walk the Duke Trail in Durham, Structure House participants talk, laugh, and focus on one another, enjoying the time to socialize and the walk. When they take our dance classes, their faces look radiant as they discover ways of combining creativity with exercise. When they experiment with weights, stair climbers, treadmills, or other kinds of equipment, they discover their own untapped potential for strength and stamina. Exercise isn't just about discipline. That's certainly an element—but it's also about learning to do something worthwhile and enjoyable.

How can you find types of exercise that *you* will enjoy? One option is to try something you've enjoyed in the past but stopped doing as you gained weight. Walking, hiking, and swimming are all good. Alternatively, you might try something altogether new. That's a great way to begin. Just tell yourself, "Okay, I'm going to *sample* this. I'm going to get a taste of the experience." Trying something even once may be sufficient to clarify whether you like it or not. Don't prejudge the outcome. Just be as present to the experience as possible. Give your full attention to it. Sometimes that first experience will show you that you'll really enjoy what you tried and that you want to come back for more.

One possibility: go to a gym with a friend. Focus on being together and supporting each other. Pick a time when you feel more comfortable—a time when it's a little less busy at the gym, perhaps. You can also try to find an environment that works for you—whether that means among people of your own gender or your general age group. Another possibility is to create your own small-scale home gym with just some basic equipment, such as free weights and a bench.

Find Some Exercise You Can *Afford*

Sometimes people tell me, "I want to exercise, but I can't afford a gym or a personal trainer." Affordability is a legitimate concern. Some trainers, clubs, and gyms *are* expensive. But costly, high-end options aren't the only ones. Many other possibilities are available—some at low cost, some entirely for free.

Consider these inexpensive options:

- Walking has no cost, and you can do it in any safe neighborhood.
- Aerobic walking, power walking, and hiking offer other no-cost options.
- YMCAs, YWCAs, Jewish community centers, and municipal community centers exist in most cities and many towns.
- Playing music at home and dancing is a convenient, no-cost option.
- Exercise videos and DVDs are widely available for purchase or rental.
- Dyna-Bands and other inexpensive equipment can provide options for resistance and strength training.
- Many communities schedule fitness classes at the local high school or community college.

Consider Other Options

These are just a few inexpensive possibilities. If your budget allows you a little more leeway, here are some other options that may involve participation in a class:

- Gyrokinesis
- Low-impact step aerobics and kickboxing

- Pilates
- Seated exercise and conditioning
- Stretching and toning
- T'ai chi and martial arts
- Weight training
- Water exercise
- Yoga

Remember: Even a Little Exercise Is Better than None

Little by little is better than fits and starts. If you build steadily but consistently over the long term, you're more likely to reach your goal of greater fitness and better health than if you proceed without creating a foundation. So first, create a foundation. Do some kind of activity consistently. Challenge yourself little by little. Gradually work your way up to greater challenges. This above all: focus on activities that you *enjoy*.

STEP 2: DEAL WITH OBSTACLES

Many people feel concerned or anxious about exercise. Perhaps you've never exercised at all, or else it's been a long time since you've done any physical activity. Perhaps you feel self-conscious about how you'll look while exercising at a gym or in some other public place, such as a park. Perhaps you simply feel that exercise will be too difficult, too time-consuming, or too uncomfortable. These are all common concerns. Read over the list below and check all the issues that bother you.

[ ] I don't have time.
[ ] I'm not motivated/I can't maintain motivation.
[ ] I've never exercised before.
[ ] I don't have the energy.
[ ] I don't have family support.
[ ] I feel embarrassed.
[ ] I'll worry about the weather/I dislike being out in bad weather.

[ ] I don't have any equipment.

[ ] I feel sick/I worry I'll get sick.

[ ] I'll dislike the discomfort.

[ ] I worry about falling.

[ ] I don't want to sweat so much.

[ ] I have low self-confidence.

[ ] I'll get bored.

[ ] The results will be too slow.

[ ] I travel too much.

[ ] I won't have any companionship while exercising.

[ ] I worry about injury or reinjury.

[ ] My work will interfere with exercise.

[ ] I won't enjoy it.

[ ] I worry about pain.

[ ] I'm concerned about criticism from other people.

[ ] I have physical limitations.

[ ] I think I'll develop friction rashes or other skin problems.

[ ] I'm worried I'll have trouble breathing.

These are all concerns that people have expressed at Structure House—obstacles that they feel prevent them from starting and maintaining an exercise program. Some people tell me that they want to check every item! Other people have specific concerns or clusters of concerns that stand out among all the others. These may be physical concerns (injury, discomfort) or emotional concerns (self-consciousness, boredom). If there's an aspect of exercise that you find challenging or threatening, it's important for you to acknowledge how you're feeling. At the same time, there are pretty straightforward solutions to each of these concerns. Here's how I'd summarize these obstacles and their solutions:

OBSTACLE	SOLUTION
I don't have time.	Almost everyone can fit some sort of exercise program into his or her schedule.

OBSTACLE	SOLUTION
I'm not motivated/I can't maintain motivation.	Most people find that their motivation increases as they get more involved in an exercise program.
I've never exercised before.	Many people haven't exercised, either—but they find they're pleasantly surprised once they get started.
I don't have the energy.	Energy usually increases once you start exercising.
I don't have family support.	You can find support from friends and others.
I feel embarrassed.	Your embarrassment will probably decrease once you experience the benefits of exercise.
I'll worry about the weather/I dislike being out in bad weather.	Many kinds of exercise can be done indoors.
I don't have any equipment.	You can use equipment at a gym or purchase low-cost equipment for home use.
I feel sick/I worry I'll get sick.	Exercise will probably increase your physical well-being, and it may help strengthen your resistance to illness.
I'll dislike the discomfort.	Discomfort can be managed and, if you proceed carefully, is usually outweighed by feelings of increased well-being.
I worry about falling.	Many kinds of exercise involve only minimal risks of falling.
I don't want to sweat so much.	Water aerobics, swimming, and other forms of aquatic exercise will eliminate this issue.

OBSTACLE	SOLUTION
I have low self-confidence.	Your self-confidence will increase as you start exercising and experience the benefits.
I'll get bored.	So many kinds of exercise exist that you can avoid or manage boredom.
The results will be too slow.	Slow-but-steady results are best, and improvements are often evident more quickly than you'd expect.
I travel too much.	Many kinds of exercise are possible while "on the go," and exercise facilities are increasingly available in hotels and elsewhere.
I won't have any companionship while exercising.	You can often find "exercise buddies" as you start to exercise.
I worry about injury or reinjury.	If you proceed carefully, the risks of injury are minimal; also, regular exercise will actually help you avoid injury as your strength, stamina, and flexibility improve.
My work will interfere with exercise.	Exercise is often feasible even for the busiest people.
I won't enjoy it.	Almost everyone enjoys some sort of exercise once you identify the kind that's right for you.
I worry about pain.	Careful planning and gradual building of skills will eliminate or minimize most kinds of pain.

OBSTACLE	SOLUTION
I'm concerned about criticism from other people.	You'll probably be less concerned about others once you experience the benefits of exercise; also, you may realize that others are paying less attention than you first thought!
I have physical limitations.	Exercise programs can be adapted to physical limitations.
I think I'll develop friction rashes or other skin problems.	Rashes can be minimized.
I'm worried I'll have trouble breathing.	With good medical advice and careful planning, you can avoid most breathing problems; in addition, exercise will generally help you increase your respiratory strength.

Now rank the top three obstacles that you've selected from the list above. Write them on the lines below. Beside the words you've written, write how you plan to overcome these obstacles.

Obstacle 1

_____

_____

Obstacle 2

_____

_____

Obstacle 3

_____

_____

Now let's consider some of the obstacles that people mention most often. I'll also suggest ways to overcome these obstacles.

"I Don't Have Time"

Everyone is busy these days, and it *is* hard to find time for exercise. But there's always a little time available—five minutes here, ten minutes there. If you don't have time for a full exercise program, you can still intentionally park a little farther from your office building or workplace when you arrive for work, then walk that extra distance. You can take a flight of stairs rather than ride the elevator. You can get up and stretch during TV commercials. All of those bits of exercise add up during the day. By moving a little more rather than a little less, you can gain strength and stamina.

Here are some other activities that you can do a little at a time.

- Walk your dog (or someone else's).
- Park farther away rather than closer when shopping, arriving at work, or visiting a friend.
- Get up to adjust the TV or CD player rather than using the remote.
- Do yard work.
- Get involved in leisure activities like bowling, badminton, croquet, etc.
- Choose your sedentary time carefully.

"I've Never Exercised Before"

People sometimes tell me that because they've never exercised in the past, even the idea of getting started is a challenge. Well, it *is* a challenge. But you don't have to run a marathon or compete in the Olympics. Just start small and see what happens. Walk around the block. Put on some music and dance. Change the pattern of your activities. The more exercise you can incorporate into your life, the easier it'll become. You've made other changes in your life; you've overcome other challenges. Think back and consider how you've mastered other difficulties in the past; then try to use that same openness to add some exercise to your routine.

"I Don't Have the Energy"

Given your busy schedule, exercise may seem the last thing you want to do. That's understandable. However, *lack* of exercise may be part of your fatigue. My recommendation: try what I call "the five-minute rule." When it's time to exercise, promise yourself you'll do it for five minutes. Then decide whether to continue or not only after reaching that milestone. Let's consider walking as an example. You feel tired, but you tell yourself you'll walk for just five minutes. I'll bet that once you walk for those five minutes, you'll feel good enough to keep going. Five minutes have let you warm up; your body feels better now; and you're feeling pretty positive about the whole experience. So you'll probably decide to walk another five minutes—or ten, or fifteen, or maybe longer. And if you decide to quit instead, you can at least say, "I did five minutes today." That's good in its own right.

"I'll Get Bored"

There's no question that if you do the same thing over and over—whether exercise or anything else—you'll get bored. But several easy steps can help solve this problem. One step is to vary your routine. (More on the options shortly.) Another is to pick exercise activities that show your progress. I urge you to experiment and set yourself gradual, progressive challenges. This may mean trying a new activity, using different kinds of equipment, trying out a different routine, or getting a new source of advice. So many options are available these days. Sample the many kinds of exercise machines. Take an aerobics class. Alternate cardiovascular workouts with weight training. Try out yoga, Pilates, or Gyrokinesis. Any activity that you like and can do safely will perk you up and help to keep your mind and body alert.

"I Won't Enjoy It"

Well, maybe you won't. But, as the saying goes, you won't know till you try it. I see the current state of exercise and fitness as a huge supermarket: you can find anything you want. If you aren't sure *what* you want, just look around at the available "merchandise." Visiting a gym or your local Y will give you all sorts of ideas. Many facilities will allow you a free visit to try the equipment, observe classes, talk with trainers, and ask a lot of questions. Exercise CDs and DVDs also provide an inexpensive, low-risk option for learning about different types of exercise and trying out the routines. One Structure House participant told me, "I want to try Pilates, but I don't know if I'm going to like it." But she *did* try it, and the next thing she knew she felt "hooked" and was taking a weekly class.

"I Have Physical Limitations"

This is a genuine concern. As I stated in Chapter 2, it's important—crucial, in fact—that you get a full medical exam before starting any exercise program. Raise any and all concerns with your primary care physician. Rule out cardiovascular, endocrine, and joint problems. Have your physician recommend the right level of exercise for your current state of health. If you have specific health problems, get them treated as soon as possible. Select your activities with care. Then proceed with the exercise program that your doctor recommends.

The bottom line: It's okay to be concerned about these obstacles, but I hope you'll be open-minded, too, and realize that all of them can be addressed. No matter what worries you may feel, there will be some kind of exercise program that will meet your needs, address your weight issues, and improve your health.

STEP 3: BOOST YOUR MOTIVATION

Of the various obstacles to exercise that people mention, the most common is probably motivation. This issue also affects even people who are committed to exercise but find it a challenge anyway. For these reasons, I'd like to address motivation as a separate step in our six-step process.

Think Positive!

My long-term goal for you is for you to be able to say, "I *like* to exercise, I'm *excited* when I exercise, and I'm *fortunate* to be able to exercise." Even people who have held off exercising for years often say very upbeat things about how exercise makes them feel. Here are just a few comments among the many positive comments that Structure House participants have made to me and members of the staff in recent years:

- "The best part is that when I'm finished, I feel I've really accomplished something."
- "I'm so proud because I did a mile this morning on my walk."
- "Now I find I can work out in bursts rather than in one big slog. I can work out for fif-

teen minutes three times a day. Half hour twice a day, or something. That's very encouraging to me."

- "I used to hate it, but now I love it."
- "It's sort of a natural high when I finish."
- "I like things that you can measure, so I'm picking types of exercise that I can do that way."

A lot of people have positive feelings about exercise. Maybe you do, too. If so, write down your own positive comments and put them up where you can see them easily and often. Write down, "When I exercise . . ." and then add what you feel. "I feel better," "I feel happier," "I feel less stressed," "I feel more energetic," "I feel less tired," "I'm proud"—whatever. Putting up these affirmations will remind you of why you're making the effort. You can wake up in the morning and say, "I want to feel good today. I want to feel a sense of accomplishment. I want to feel proud of myself. Therefore, I'm lucky to be able to exercise, which will help me in these ways." This kind of language helps you to see exercise not as a chore but as something that's positive—something that makes both your body and your mind feel good.

Set Goals

Another way to boost your motivation is to set specific goals for yourself. Rather than seeing exercise as a huge all-or-nothing effort, you should set both short-term and long-term goals. It's important for your goals to be *attainable* and *measurable*. If your goal is to walk for twenty minutes on the treadmill, start by aiming for five or ten. Your short-term goal might be to increase the time by two minutes each week. If you're walking for ten minutes this week, shoot for twelve minutes next week, then fourteen, then sixteen, until you've reached the goal of twenty.

If you're setting a yearlong goal, make a timeline. Specify your year-end goal. Then calculate what's realistic for the midpoint at six months. How are you going to break those first six months into monthly goals? From there, figure out your weekly goals. This process will take some work initially, but it'll pay off in the long run because it's going to provide a constant sense of accomplishment. You'll see the results and the benefits every week. Then, before you know it, you'll reach your intermediate goal and, eventually, your long-term goal.

Other Strategies for Staying Motivated

- Keep your "Dear Me" letter handy and refer to it often, reminding yourself why you are making positive lifestyle changes.
- Approach your lifestyle changes as if it were a business. What is your strategic plan? Plan ahead.
- Set small, realistic goals, and reevaluate them periodically.
- Keep a record of your activities.
- Keep a record of your accomplishments that don't have anything to do with your weight. (Examples: You are now able to climb a flight of stairs without getting out of breath; you can now cross your legs, which makes tying your shoes easier; you weren't able to hold the hair dryer up long enough to dry your hair, and now you can.)
- Choose a time for exercise that fits into your lifestyle.
- Progress gradually. Increase first frequency and duration, then intensity.
- Keep a gym bag loaded with exercise clothes in your car.
- Add activity into your daily life in little ways (do yard work, clean house, park farther away from your destination, walk the dog).
- Avoid "black-and-white" thinking.
- Try a new activity—a dance class, yoga class, or walking club.
- Don't use your obstacles as an excuse.
- Hire a personal trainer.
- Join a class.
- Get your friends or spouse involved as your support system.
- Use daily affirmations and visualization to keep you motivated.
- Attach meaning to your exercise (on a hike, for instance: you're communing with nature, you're spending quality time with your spouse, you're keeping in contact with friends).

Make a Commitment

Another way to boost your motivation is to make a commitment. You can simply tell yourself you're going to exercise, of course, and perhaps that's a good enough commitment for your purposes. On the other hand, a lot of people find that putting the commitment in writing—a "contract with yourself," so to speak—is more durable, something you'll see on the wall, think about, remember, and act upon more readily than if you just make a vague promise to yourself.

Here's a "Commitment to Exercise" that many Structure House participants have found useful.

My Commitment to Exercise

I have decided to adopt a healthier lifestyle in the area of exercise and fitness!

My goal in the next three months is (be specific) _____
_____

And I *will* accomplish this by _____
_____

Trying to do everything all at once can be overwhelming. Also, I may injure myself or get discouraged if I move too fast. For these reasons, I'm going to take *small steps* in the right direction each week.

Step 1 (Tomorrow): _____
_____

Step 2 (By next week): _____
_____

Step 3 (By next month): _____
_____

I will measure my progress by: _____

I am going to enlist the support and encouragement of: _____

In other areas of my life I've demonstrated the ability to get things done, and I've overcome challenges to make this happen. I can use those same skills to improve my personal fitness.

Obstacles   Solutions

_____   _____

_____   _____

_____   _____

Rewards or incentives for achieving my goals: _____
_____

I have the power to choose a healthy lifestyle. Even though I'll encounter challenges and setbacks, I can make these important changes. I'm committed to making a difference in my health and developing a physically active lifestyle that works for me.

Signed: _____   Date: _____
Witness: _____

STEP 4: UNDERSTAND THE THREE ELEMENTS OF EXERCISE

At this point you may protest, "Okay, this sounds great—but I don't know *how* to reach these goals. I don't know enough about exercise to create a healthy program."

Don't worry. I can provide you with an outline for a good, safe exercise program, and I'll also suggest some resources that can help you customize the program in more detail.

Here's the core issue.

The American College of Sports Medicine (ACSM) recommends a

combination of three types of physical activity for people interested in losing weight: *cardiovascular (aerobic) exercise; strength training;* and *flexibility training.* These three forms of exercise complement one another, and each is important in its own right. I urge you to use all three kinds and not get carried away with any one of them at the expense of the others. Let's have a look at them one by one.

Exercise Component 1: Cardiovascular (Aerobic) Training

Cardiovascular exercise ("cardio" for short) is continuous movement that uses large muscle groups. It's also referred to as *aerobic* activity. Some examples of cardio include walking or jogging, walking or jogging on a treadmill, using a stationary bike; using an elliptical trainer or a stair stepper; and doing low-impact aerobics, water aerobics, or water walking. All of these activities use your major large-muscle groups. The standard recommendation is that you do thirty to sixty minutes of cardiovascular activity at least five days a week.

Here's why this kind of exercise is important. The heart is a muscle that needs to be strengthened (just like any other muscle). To do so, you need to "load" it beyond its normal capacity—that is, to push it beyond its normal limits to build strength, which is called *overload*. The standard measurement for overload is 60 to 80 percent of *maximal overload*. Maximal overload is a factor of age. Biologically speaking, your heart slows down as you age. A formula derived through research has proved to be a fairly accurate standard measure of heart rate. For this reason, the "training effect" or "overload principle" means that you need to push beyond normal limits into the 60 to 80 percent of maximal heart rate per minute.

How do you know how to reach that 60 to 80 percent zone? That's an important subject, so let's explore it.

Your heart rate is the number of times your heart beats per minute. Your heart rate measures how hard your body is working (what we call the *intensity*) during your cardiovascular workout. Beginners should focus on exercising so that they stay in the lower end of the range. As you proceed with training, you can aim higher within the range.

Following is a chart that shows your age-adjusted heart rate range. You should aim for a level of exertion that places your heart rate within the range for your age.[1]

Age	Heart Rate Range
30	95–160
35	92–157
40	90–153
45	87–148
50	85–144
55	82–140
60	80–136
65	77–131

As you exercise, check your pulse periodically. Using the index and middle fingers of one hand, gently press on either the radial artery (on your wrist at the base of the thumb) or the carotid artery (on your neck, to the side of the larynx). Count your pulse for 15 seconds (the first pulse you hear counts as zero). Multiply that number by 4. The number you get is your one-minute heart rate.

Alternatively, you can use a heart rate monitor, a small, watchlike device whose digital readout will display your heart rate at any given moment. These monitors are easy to use, reliable, and accurate in indicating the intensity of your exercise and the rate of perceived exertion. They can easily help you understand how your body responds to physically demanding effort; some models have alarms that can be programmed to signal when you're either too high or too low in relation to your target heart rate.

Cardiovascular exercise has several benefits. Over time, your heart muscle becomes stronger as you train. Your heart gains the ability to pump more blood per beat, which carries more nutrients and oxygen to your muscles and also carries away more waste products. As your heart becomes stronger, it doesn't have to beat as fast, thus using less energy and preserving energy for other activities.

Another benefit of cardiovascular training is the potential for weight loss. Aerobic (low-intensity) activity utilizes an energy system that burns fat as fuel. Anaerobic (high-intensity) activity uses more carbohydrates as fuel. The more intense the exercise, the fewer fats and oxygen are used. Higher intensity levels mean that the body has to produce quicker energy. The body accommodates this need with an energy system that uses carbohydrates as energy, and it undergoes a different process, thus supplying the muscles with the energy they need without having to wait for the oxygen to be delivered from the heart. The lower the intensity level of the exercise, the more fats are used as fuel.

What I'm describing has two implications:

- First, the approximate level of overload to the heart muscle can help improve the cardiovascular system to achieve optimal endurance levels and a more energetic, healthier lifestyle.
- Second, the appropriate level of overload or intensity can help you maintain an efficient energy system and metabolic rate to utilize fats and improve your physical appearance.

You can meet both of these goals better if you monitor your heartbeats per minute and maintain the recommended 60 to 80 percent range per minute.

Here are a few other important recommendations:

- **Start slowly.** The duration of your exercise may only be a minute or two when you first start out; then you can gradually increase your time by 1 or 2 minutes each time you exercise until you can exercise continuously for at least 20 minutes. Begin gently and work up to a higher level of activity. Pushing too hard too fast may risk injury and frustration. Perhaps you'll start by doing 5 minutes in the morning, 5 minutes in the afternoon, and 5 minutes in the evening. Making small but steady progress is far better than overdoing it.

- **Warm up before and cool down after your activity for at least five to ten minutes.** Warming up will ensure that you're supplying enough blood to all your working muscles. Cooling down will prevent *blood pooling,* a process that can leave you feeling light-headed if you stop exercising too suddenly.

- **If you perform cardiovascular activity five or more days a week, alternate weight-bearing with non-weight-bearing exercise** (i.e., walk one day, then ride a bike or swim the next day). This is called "cross training." It's important because it lets your body rest from one activity as you do the other, and it also keeps your body alert and awake. I'll have more to say about weight-bearing and non-weight-bearing activities in a moment.

Exercise Component 2: Strength (Resistance) Training

Strength training is exercising with resistance for the purpose of strengthening the musculoskeletal system. This component of exercise focuses on a different set of goals than cardio workouts do: it increases your muscular strength, muscular endurance, tendon and ligament tensile strength, and bone strength. As a result of these benefits, you'll be stronger overall; you'll be able to deal more easily with physical challenges, such as walking, climbing stairs, and carrying loads; and you'll tire less easily. Strong muscles help support joints and increase structural integrity, which means that your joints can handle stress more efficiently and are less susceptible to injury. Even four weeks of training will produce a noticeable difference in your overall strength. In addition, stronger muscles require more energy and thus utilize more calories, which may have a side effect of helping you lose weight.

Generally speaking, you should do strength training two or three days per week, with 48 hours between strength training sessions. Exercises focus on eight to ten muscles at a time, with 8 to 15 repetitions of each exercise in each set and one or two sets of each exercise. Strength training can be done with any of the following kinds of equipment and techniques:

- Free weights (dumbbells or a barbell)
- Weight machines
- Dyna-Bands
- Your own body weight (push-ups, abdominal crunches, etc.)
- Body sculpting
- Stretch and tone
- Pilates
- Core conditioning
- Resist-A-Ball

Here are some general recommendations for strength training:

- **Timing.** Expect your strength training routine to take 20 to 45 minutes. When you first start strength training, one set is enough for the first few weeks. Gradually add repetitions first before adding another set.

- **Intensity.** Use enough weight to fatigue the muscle within 8 to 15 repetitions. If you can do 15 repetitions easily, the weight is too light. If you can't do at least 8 repetitions, the weight is too heavy. Once you can do more than 15 repetitions, increase the weight to the next increment available and decrease your repetitions accordingly.

- **Variety.** Each muscle group will require a different weight to fatigue the muscle. Your muscles should feel fatigued after you complete up to 15 repetitions. Rest that muscle group for 30 to 90 seconds before starting the second set.

- **Frequency of workouts.** Train two or three times per week, with at least 48 hours between sessions. One set with appropriate weight is sufficient. Two sets return a little more benefit. Rest between sets. Do not strength train the same muscle groups on two consecutive days; your muscles need a chance to rest.

- **Exercise speed.** Slow and controlled is best. For example, take 2 seconds to lift and 4 seconds to lower the weight.

- **Breathe.** Don't hold your breath. Exhale on the exertion (resistance effort) and inhale on the release.

Exercise Component 3: Flexibility Training

Flexibility training improves your ability to move muscles and joints in their full range of motion. Many people do flexibility exercises on the days they're not doing strength training; the ideal goal is about two to three days per week.

Typical activities for flexibility training include:

- Stretching for flexibility
- Yoga
- T'ai chi
- Stretch and tone

At Structure House, our exercise instructors offer these general recommendations to enhance flexibility:

- **Stretch each major muscle group three to five times, holding each stretch for a minimum of 20 seconds.** You may find that you prefer stretching longer. Twenty seconds gets your muscle to a point to where it relaxes and allows your body to stretch a little bit further.

- **Stretch just enough until you feel the muscle tension.** Muscle tension should decrease while you are stretching; if it doesn't, you're stretching too far.

- **Don't hold your breath.** While you're stretching, keep breathing. You will find that, as with strength training, breathing will help your body to relax. Use your breath to allow your body to focus and to work effectively.

- **Don't "lock" your joints.** That will risk hyperextending, which can lead to injury.

- **Don't bounce.** Sports physiologists have determined that bouncing, too, increases the risk of injury. Avoid stretching in ways that hurt. If you feel pain, consult your physician.

Listen to Your Body

Finally, I want to emphasize a critical aspect of exercise: No matter what exercise program appeals to you, you need to listen to your body. Each person's body is unique. Even if you have a well-trained, thoughtful exercise instructor, *you* should tune in to the cues and warning signals you're receiving from your body. Ignoring these cues and signals may result in stress or injury. This is especially true if you're overweight, since your body is already physiologically stressed.

Listening to your body may be more difficult than you think. First of all, you have to learn to tune in to the signals you're receiving, and tuning in like this takes time and practice. In addition, some exercise environments, such as classes, may prompt you to feel a sense of peer pressure. You may also feel your *own* expectations about what you want to happen—or how quickly you want it to. If so, you may neglect to notice what your body needs. You may tend to ignore fatigue or pain. You may become obsessed with a "No pain, no gain" mentality. In doing so, you may risk injuring yourself even more.

Here's an important truth: your body will make requests to you about what it needs and doesn't need. If you can consider a little twinge or ache as a request, you can evaluate what you're doing to your body. Maybe you'll slow down. Maybe you'll move more carefully. You need to be fully *present* to yourself. Being present will help you avoid overdoing, fatiguing yourself, and risking injury. Listening to your body will help you be *consistent*, which is a better approach than overdoing anyway.

STEP 5: DESIGN AN EXERCISE SCHEDULE

If you can do cardio exercise, strength training, and flexibility training, you'll provide your body with the combination of activities most likely to improve your overall health and contribute to your weight loss efforts. It's important to balance these forms of exercise in a program that avoids missing opportunities but also avoids overtraining. The general goals are the same for most programs:

- **Cardiovascular/aerobic exercise:** 30 to 60 minutes on most days of the week at a moderate intensity.
- **Strength training:** Two to three times per week—one to two sets of 8 to 15 reps working eight to ten muscle groups.
- **Flexibility exercises:** At least three times per week. (You should also stretch every time you exercise.)

What's the best way to assemble these goals into a program? I'd like to suggest four options.

Option 1: Plan Your Schedule on Your Own

The simplest option is to design your own schedule. This option has the advantage of being inexpensive; on the other hand, it has the disadvantage of lacking outside guidance, which may save you time and trouble in the long run. If you decide to plan your own schedule, consider these guidelines[2]:

Cut down on

- watching TV
- playing computer games
- sitting for more than 30 minutes

2 to 3 days a week

- **Leisure activity:** golf, bowling, softball, yard work
- **Flexibility/strength:** stretching/yoga, push-ups, curl ups, weight lifting

3 to 5 days a week

- **Aerobic exercise** (30+ minutes): brisk walking, cross-country skiing, bicycling, swimming
- **Recreational exercise** (30+ minutes): soccer, hiking, basketball, tennis, martial arts, dancing

Every day

- Walk the dog
- Walk to the store or mailbox
- Take longer routes
- Work in your garden
- Take the stairs instead of the elevator
- Park car farther away from your destination
- Make extra steps in your day

Following these guidelines, you can create your own exercise plan using the chart on page 157 to photocopy and fill out:

My Exercise Plan

	SUNDAY	MONDAY	TUESDAY	WEDNESDAY	THURSDAY	FRIDAY	SATURDAY
Aerobic activity **When & Where** Frequency: 5 days Time: 20–60 min.							
Strength training Frequency: 2 to 3 days Time: 30 to 60 min.							
Flexibility Frequency: 2 to 3 days Time: 5 or 10–15 min.							

In addition, you should consider some other factors carefully if you decide to design your own exercise program:

Purchase Equipment Carefully

If you decide to purchase equipment for home use, I urge you to follow these guidelines:

- Shop at a reputable fitness equipment store, bicycle shop, or dealer.
- Work with a well-trained staff that knows the equipment and can explain all the features.
- Be prepared to try each piece of equipment—don't rush to do anything without a "test drive" first.
- Wear exercise clothing and use each machine for ten minutes to see if it is comfortable. Try various speeds, settings, resistance levels, inclines, and so forth. Is it stable? Will it last as you become more fit? What is the maximum weight capacity?
- Determine if there's a weight restriction. Most home equipment is safe for a user up to 350 pounds. Equipment for commercial use (in a health club) often has much higher weight restrictions.
- Ask about a money-back guarantee or a trial period so that if the equipment doesn't meet your expectations you can return it.
- Check in advance with *Consumer Reports,* as this publication (and Web site) often reviews home exercise equipment. Do your homework!
- Before purchasing, ask:
  - Does the company sell used or refurbished equipment?
  - Does it offer a lease-before-purchase arrangement?
  - Is there a maintenance contract? Who in your area can fix the equipment if you have any problems with it?
  - Is there a warranty, and how long does it last?
  - Does the company deliver and/or assemble equipment?
- Know how to use all the features before you purchase any equipment.

Option 2: Join a Gym or Health Club

Maybe you prefer not to "fly solo." You may not feel confident of your ability to set up a program yourself, or you worry that you'll have trouble following it without other people's company or encouragement. There's nothing wrong with wanting some guidance or companionship. Fortunately, many options exist that can satisfy these needs. Private health clubs are one option. Community centers (YMCAs, YWCAs, Jewish community centers, and other similar organizations) are another.

In addition to finding resources that fit your budget, here are some other factors you should consider as you select a gym or health club:

- **Location.** The club should be no more than 10 to 15 minutes from home or work. If the club is too far away, it will be difficult to stick to your exercise regimen.
- **Classes and equipment.** Does the facility have a pool, aerobics classes for your fitness level, Pilates, yoga, group strength training? Are the classes on the days and at the times when you can attend?
- **Staff.** Are the trainers certified by reputable organizations?
- **Hours.** Will you have access to equipment and classes when your schedule permits?
- **Trial membership.** Will the club or gym allow you a free day- or weeklong pass to try out the facility?
- **Amenities.** Does the facility offer massages, towel service, lockers, and other services?
- **Atmosphere.** How does the club or gym feel to you? Visit the club during the hours you are most likely to attend to see how crowded it is, what type of music is played, and what type of people go there when you are most likely going to be there. Is the music to your liking, particularly with respect to the type and loudness?
- **Members.** Will you fit in there or be uncomfortable? Are people of a variety of ages and fitness levels present? If not, the club may cater to a particular age group or style. Is that a group or style whose presence you'll find comfortable?

Option 3: Hire a Personal Trainer

One of the best options for designing an exercise program is to get advice from a personal trainer. It's true that hiring a trainer can be expensive over a long period of time; a short-term consultation, however, can provide you with a lot of information and tailor-made suggestions for a modest cash outlay. Even a couple of sessions can clarify a lot of issues, ease your anxieties, and give you expert recommendations about the equipment you need and the procedures you should follow. Many personal trainers will help you become self-sufficient. In addition, a personal trainer can boost your motivation, help you spot problems before they develop, strengthen your confidence, and understand your body's signals. Following this initial consultation, you can proceed on your own or, ideally, check in with the trainer every few months to clarify issues over the long term.

To simplify the task of finding and consulting with a personal trainer, here are some questions to ask:

- **Is the trainer certified? If so, by whom?** The best certifications are from the ACSM (American College of Sports Medicine), ACE (American Council on Exercise), and NSCA (National Strength and Conditioning Association). To find an ACSM-certified professional in your area, visit www.acsm.org/certification/FORMS/online_locator .asp. (The ACSM's certifications are "Health and Fitness Instructor" and "Exercise Specialist.") To find an ACE professional in your area, visit www.acefitness.org/profreg/index.cfm. (The ACE's certifications are "Personal Trainer" and "Clinical Exercise Specialist.")

- **What type of experience does the trainer have?** Ask for references.

- **Does the trainer have liability insurance?** Ask to see the certificate of coverage. Also, consider asking to see a written copy of the trainer's business policies.

- **Do you have special needs?** If so, make sure the trainer knows how to handle them. (Does your trainer know the difference in how to train a sixty-year-old as compared to a twenty-five-year-old?)

- **What does the trainer charge?** Payment can vary considerably (depending on the club or gym, the trainer's experience, and the nature of the consultation, such as whether the trainer comes to your home or not). Some trainers offer discounts for multiple sessions. (Caveat: Most packages have an expiration date.)

- **What is the trainer's fitness philosophy? What is his or her personality like?** Is this someone you feel you can work with? If you aren't sure, pay for one session first.

See if you feel that you can develop a rapport. Determine if the trainer can support your goals and needs.

Option 4: Do "Nontraditional" Exercise

Finally, I want to suggest kinds of exercise that are less traditional or less organized than what I've described so far. These are ways of exercising that can supplement more systematic programs, but they can also be substantial in their own right. Many of the ideas I'll mention are ordinary activities that we tend to avoid just because we have "laborsaving devices" or services that save us the trouble of exerting ourselves. A better idea: Get out there and *move*. Here are some suggestions.

- Run easy errands on foot.
- Walk the dog.
- Work in your garden.
- Park farther away from rather than closer to the store or wherever else you're going.
- Put on a CD or the radio and dance.
- Join a mall-walking club.
- Buy a pedometer and track your progress.

You can do almost anything. Just put motion into your life.

PART III

STAY STRUCTURED

Maintain
the Structure House
Weight Loss Plan

Stay Structured Away from Home: Eating Well and Losing Weight in Restaurants and on the Road

"I've found it remarkably easy to lose weight away from Structure House if I just do what I'm supposed to do. Eating out a lot (which I do) makes things difficult but not insurmountable. I went on a two-and-a-half-week road trip in July and ended up gaining only a pound the entire time."

—Anella

"To stay structured . . . I confine myself to about five safe eating places. I know that the choice I make at each place is safe and healthy."

—Kate

If eating at home presents a variety of opportunities and risks, the same holds true for eating away from home. In public, you have fewer chances for succumbing to food habits—sneaking snacks, nibbling as you prepare your meals, and so forth—but you also have far less control over when and what you eat. In addition, many restaurants cook with highly energy-dense ingredients, serve massive portions, and offer all sorts of high-calorie temptations.

In fact, most people feel that they do a better job of staying Structured at home. However, others can actually do better in a restaurant. At home they're cooking, serving, and cleaning up for the whole family. Food cues may be far more abundant and tempting at home. "Closet eaters," for instance, may stay Structured more easily in restaurants because they do their heavy eating when they're alone. When they're in a restaurant, they don't have access to the refrigerator and to second servings. Nevertheless, most people have more difficulty *controlling* their food intake in a restaurant than they do at home. You may arrive when it's already past your usual eating time, so you're extrahungry; you smell many enticing aromas in the air; and you read the menu and all those tempting descriptions like "tender morsels cut from the heart of the filet, cooked to perfection, and smothered in Madeira sauce." Then, once you've ordered, you have the bread basket and appetizers to contend with. And after the entrées, you face the challenges of coping with the dessert menu or, worse yet, "temptation on wheels": the dessert cart.

How can you respond to these situations and still stay Structured? If you know what to expect, strategize ahead of time, and follow these four straightforward tasks, it's not as difficult as you may imagine.

TASK 1: LEARN TO STAY STRUCTURED IN RESTAURANTS

Although there are advantages for some people, others may find that eating in restaurants creates some special challenges. It's hard to plan ahead. There's the potential for social pressure from your dining companions. It's easy to make impulsive choices. And options may be more restricted than at home. It's also tempting to decide, "Okay, I've been Structured at home, now I can let loose and reward myself," or "I can't help it if I get unstructured—I'm just a guest here."

Are you reluctant to preplan your meals before you arrive at the restaurant? Perhaps eating out is part of your business entertaining, or perhaps you go out only for social occasions. You may be thinking, "Wait just a minute! Preplanning isn't realistic. I frequently go out to eat, but I don't necessarily know where I'm going to be, which friends or coworkers I'll be with, or which restaurant we're going to visit." I realize that under circumstances like these, Structured Eating in restaurants may seem like a daunting task.

Rest easy. You can master these situations and use them to your advantage. How? Let me tell you.

First of all, keep this core principle in mind: *Any situation can be Structured*. Granted, some are easier to Structure than others, but all can be adapted in one way or another to the Structure House approach. This chapter will give you a wide range of tools to make this task easier.

Second, when you plan your food choices, you're more likely to choose foods on the basis of nourishment rather than when "impulse buying." If you wait until you reach the restaurant to start coping with all the food cues that these places present—aromas, bread baskets, buffets, dessert carts, and all the rest—you're more likely to choose foods for reasons that have nothing to do with nourishment. You'll probably resort to Unstructured Eating.

Keep in mind that even "winging it" involves making choices. Let's say you go to a Tex-Mex theme restaurant with some friends. You decide simply to follow your whims and hope for the best—but from the start you're making impulsive decisions. "Oooh, look at the guacamole those folks at the next table are having!" you exclaim. "Let's have some, too!" Ordering the guacamole means you'll need lots of salty fried tortilla chips, of course, so you ask for a basket of those to accompany the dip. Soon you're thirsty, so you order a huge margarita. And the entrees? "I want the beef enchiladas," you announce. "In fact, make that the enchilada special"—which, as you might have guessed, comes with refried beans, lots of grated cheese, a rather oily rice pilaf, and a little basket of flour tortillas. By the time you've eaten all this food, you're stuffed. But that doesn't stop you and your friends from ordering *sopaipillas* for dessert—puffy triangles of deep-fried dough dipped in honey!

So did you make decisions about your meal? Of course. You just didn't create any Structure as you made them.

A better approach is planning ahead. You phone the Tex-Mex place during off-hours in advance to check out what's available. Before you even step into the restaurant, you have an overview of what will fit the Structured approach. You decide in advance on grilled red snapper in *salsa roja*, a medley of sautéed squash and corn, a big salad, and a corn tortilla. When you arrive, you pass on the guacamole and chips, order the meal you've already planned, enjoy every bite, and proceed to have a splendid time with your dining companions. *Salud!*—To your health!

Ironically, some Structure House participants tell me, "I have my unhealthy meal all preplanned—every unhealthy, high-calorie thing I'm going to eat—before I ever walk into the restaurant." Well, if you can mentally preplan an *unhealthy* meal, you can certainly preplan a *healthy* one.

Staying Structured *is* possible—it just requires a little forethought. You can often nip problems in the bud by identifying fail-safe meals ahead of time with just a few phone calls to restaurants or hotels. You can develop confidence in your ability to manage restaurant eating. Follow these steps to make the process easier.

ASK YOURSELF WHY YOU'RE EATING OUT

Are you eating out to use high-calorie food as "the main event"? I hope not. A better approach: View the food as nourishment; then focus on the company of the people you're with, the restaurant's atmosphere, and the occasion itself as a source of enjoyment and entertainment. You're not at the Tex-Mex place to overeat but to enjoy the company of your friends, share a good time together, and hear the mariachis.

OBTAIN A MENU IN ADVANCE

Many restaurants have menus available that you can pick up or have faxed to you. Some restaurants will also provide detailed nutrition information about their meals. A growing number of restaurants, especially nationwide chain restaurants, now post nutritional data on the Internet. Whatever method you use to obtain the menu or other information, getting it in advance will give you a huge advantage in planning structured meals.

BE ALERT TO HIDDEN INFORMATION

Menus often contain terms that provide hidden information for what you'll encounter. If you're alert to these terms, you'll be ahead of the game.

- **Low-fat preparation terms:** "Steamed"; "broiled"; "roasted"; "poached"; "garden fresh"; "in its own juice"; "dry roasted."
- **Low-fat terms suggesting possibly high sodium content:** "Pickled"; "in cocktail sauce"; "smoked"; "in broth"; "in tomato base."
- **High-fat preparation terms:** "Buttery"; "butter sauce"; "sautéed"; "fried"; "crispy"; "braised"; "creamed"; "in its own gravy"; "au gratin"; "parmesan"; "escalloped"; "marinated"; "basted"; "prime"; "fluffy"; "tempura."

ASK QUESTIONS

What's listed on the menu is an indication of the raw materials in the kitchen, not necessarily the specific way the chefs will prepare the food. For this reason, it's worthwhile to call the restaurant ahead of time to ask some questions. Too shy? Call and ask anyway. You're offering the restaurant your business; most good restaurateurs are eager to accommodate their customers. I've heard almost countless times from Structure House participants that restaurant staffs respond helpfully to requests for nutrition information, even in big cities like New York and Los Angeles. I've also had many personal experiences of speaking with restaurant personnel and finding them earnest and responsive to my requests. The restaurant business is intensely competitive, so chefs need to please their patrons. Don't assume that personnel won't give you the help you need! And if they don't, give them a vote of no confidence by eating somewhere else. I encourage you to patronize restaurants whose owners and chefs are responsive to your concerns about nutrition.

Here are some "starters" to get your conversation under way:

- "Thanks for taking time to speak with me. I'm on a special diet, so I have a few questions about the selections you offer at your restaurant."
- "Because of some health issues, I need to check with you about how you prepare some of your dishes."
- "I have some dietary restrictions, so I'd appreciate a little information about what you serve and how you prepare certain foods."

Call during a slack time (such as the middle of the afternoon) when the staff will have time to answer your questions. Request to speak with someone who can really answer your questions, such as the chef or the manager. Most establishments will try to be helpful.

Here are some typical questions to ask.

If your time is limited—or if the person you're speaking with seems rushed—ask a few "big-picture" questions:

- I'm on a restricted diet. Do you serve any low-fat, low-sodium entrees?
- Can sauces, dressing, gravies, and condiments be served on the side?
- Can you make some entrées with certain ingredients held back or reduced in quantity?
- Can vegetables be steamed or cooked without fat or salt?
- Will diet dressing, diet drinks, sweeteners, fresh fruit, or skim milk be available?

If you have more time available, or if you are interacting with someone at the restaurant who seems unusually helpful, ask more detailed questions:

- Can portions be measured and altered in the kitchen?
- Is it possible to get meat, fish, or poultry broiled or baked with or without advance notice?
  - Is oil put on the grill before grilling meats?
  - Are meat, fish, and poultry dry broiled, baked, or grilled?
  - Are meat, fish, and poultry marinated before or after preparation? With what?
- Are there high-calorie hidden ingredients used in preparation?

- What comes on the salad?
- Are there any hidden items on the menus? For example, do entrées come garnished with cooked vegetables that aren't mentioned on menu? If so, can these items be prepared in a low-calorie manner?
- Are there high-calorie ingredients (butter, margarine, oil, mayonnaise, cheeses) used in preparation?

If you've been able to obtain the restaurant's menu before you make your phone call, your questions can be even more specific, zeroing in on particular entrees, for instance. Use your judgment about how much detail to request. A good impression of the restaurant's overall flexibility, for instance, tells you enough that you don't need to ask about every last detail about food preparation.

At the Restaurant

Here are some strategies for dealing with the restaurant itself:

- **Don't arrive superhungry.** If you show up at the restaurant way past your usual mealtime, you'll be extrahungry at precisely the time when you're confronted with the many temptations present in a restaurant.

- **Don't look at the menu.** Since you've planned your meal in advance, you don't need to consult it again. All those elaborate descriptions of the meals will complicate your efforts to stay Structured.

- **If possible, place your order first.** The person who orders first sets the tone for everyone else. If the first person orders a big appetizer and the richest entrée, everyone else will get into the spirit and do the same thing. It's harder to stick with your plan when you've heard what other people have requested. If it isn't feasible to order first, just stay as close as possible to your original plan.

- **To the greatest degree possible, eliminate food temptations.** If you're at the restaurant alone—or with a friend who's responsive to the Structured approach—you can remove certain problematic food cues, such as the bread basket. Ask the waiter not to bring it. If you're with people who want the bread, decide in advance that you'll pass. When your fellow diners have taken the bread they want, send the rest of the bread away.

Your use of these approaches will depend partly on the company you're keeping at the restaurant. If you're among close friends, you'll have more flexibility in what you do or don't do. If you're among business associates or less close friends, you'll need to be more discreet and selective in what you request or do. Keep in mind that, in general, people are increasingly respectful of others' dietary needs. You don't want to come off as a control freak, but you certainly have a right to address your nutritional and health needs.

Build a "Database" of Favorites

You probably have a limited number of favorite restaurants. Most people have a mental list of their "top five" or "top ten." For this reason, it's worthwhile to save the information you acquire about these restaurants and keep it for future use. You owe it to yourself to have the best data available—a game plan for all your favorite restaurants. Preplan meals for each of those restaurants, then save the info in an easy-access format. This format can be as low-tech as notes scribbled on 3-by-5-inch note cards or as high-tech as entries in a PDA.

Here's how you can use this information in several different settings.

- **Casual get-togethers are easy.** If you're in the company of close friends, you can be open about your special needs. Even consulting your notes on site probably won't be a problem. Many Structure House participants find that friends and relatives are supportive of their efforts to stay Structured, since they may be concerned about weight and health issues, too.

- **A more formal occasion,** such as dinner at a high-end restaurant, may require greater care in how you review your "database." This is a situation where checking your notes in advance will pay off. A phone call to the restaurant is likely to simplify the process and diminish the self-consciousness you may feel when at the table with your fellow diners.

- **Repeat visits make the whole process easier.** If you're a regular at a particular restaurant, you'll already know what's available and what you want, and the proprietors will be all the more willing to accommodate you. ("Please remember, I'd like that fish broiled, not fried.")

- **Business occasions.** Work-related restaurant visits create special concerns for many people. You may be dining with people you don't know well—or at all—and you want to be professional. At the same time, you want to stay the course with Structured Eating. The solution: to the degree possible, plan ahead. Consult your notes in advance. Interact with the restaurant staff by phone before you arrive, if possible. You don't want your nutritional needs to dominate the occasion, but those needs are, in fact, legitimate. Finding the right balance may take some experimentation. Remember: people are increasingly aware of others' nutritional needs, whether it's an issue of allergies, religious dietary restrictions, or health concerns. You probably aren't the only person at the table who has special preferences. You don't have to give up eating in restaurants. Just get savvy, get Structured, and get organized. What follows are specific recommendations for staying Structured at restaurants—first at chain restaurants; then at ethnic restaurants.

Task 2: Stay Structured at Chain Restaurants

I'm most likely to go to a chain restaurant—especially a fast-food restaurant—when I'm on a long car trip. These restaurants are everywhere, so they're often the easiest option while traveling. Their rapid spread throughout the nation presents both advantages and disadvantages.

The advantage of chain restaurants is that everything is standardized. No matter where you find an Applebee's, a Cracker Barrel, a Ruby Tuesday, or a Wendy's, you'll be dealing with the same products and the same caloric value at every individual restaurant within that particular chain. This situation can make planning meals relatively easy. Restaurants with health-oriented choices (sometimes noted on the menu as "Heart-Healthy Selections") are especially convenient on long road trips, for meals of this sort easily lend themselves to Structured Eating. The disadvantage, unfortunately, is that much of the food served at chain restaurants is high-calorie, high-fat, high-sodium fare. It's easy to go overboard and overeat. Some people feel that eating at chain restaurants offers too many temptations. But because chain restaurants are so widespread—they are now truly the "default" option throughout much of the United States—it's all the more important to understand how to cope with them.

Problem Meals and Healthy Meals

First let's look at a few numbers. What's the maximum intake of fat you should have in a whole day at different caloric levels?

- If you're on 1,200 calories, no more than 40 grams.
- If you're on 1,400 calories, no more than 47 grams.
- If you're on 1,600 calories, no more than 53 grams.

Don't get me wrong: I'm not suggesting that you count grams of fat in every single food you eat, add it up, and total it for the day. That's too complex and laborious. If you use the guidelines I've noted, though, you'll come out just fine.

Keeping these figures in mind, let's look at some healthy meals that you can find at American chain restaurants today. All of these options allow you to avoid what I call problem meals—meals that are way too high in calories, fat, sodium, or all three. Each of the following restaurants offers both good news and bad news. But by checking ahead and looking up nutrition data on the chains' Web sites, you can save yourself a lot of trouble. Not all of the restaurants I'll list currently post their data on the Web, but many do, and more and more are doing so all the time. (In the autumn of 2005, even McDonald's started providing nutrition information to customers![1])

Applebee's
A lot of chain restaurants now offer healthy choices, and they post the nutrition data for these options right on the Internet. For instance, Applebee's has a Weight Watchers menu.

Here's an example: the sizzling chicken skillet with vegetables on whole wheat tortillas. It has 360 calories, 4 grams of fat. One option is to double the vegetables. Applebee's also lists many other choices suitable to Structured Eating.

Chili's Grill & Bar Family Restaurant

This chain has what they call its Guiltless Grill menu. Of Chili's many good choices, consider the Guiltless Chicken sandwich with black beans and vegetables—490 calories, 8 grams of fat. Something else to keep in mind about Chili's: it has many Structure-friendly side dishes. (Remember, when you're staying Structured, an easy "guesstimate" is that half of the food on your plate should be vegetables; no more than a quarter of what's there should be animal protein; and no more than a quarter should be starch.)

T.G.I. Friday's

Among the several good choices at T.G.I. Friday's is the Barbecue Jack chicken with black beans and corn salsa, rice, grilled vegetables, and steamed broccoli—500 calories, 10 grams of fat. Another is bruschetta tilapia—whitefish topped with tomato basil salsa and balsamic glaze, served with steamed herb rice and broccoli—500 calories, 10 grams of fat.

Ruby Tuesday

On this chain's "Smart Eating" menu, a good bet is the white chicken chili, which is an appetizer you can eat as a main dish. There are also lots of vegetable sides to go with it. You could get the grilled chicken seasoned with peppercorns—209 calories, 5 grams of fat—with fresh steamed broccoli and a side Caesar salad. The total for the meal: 458 calories, 23 grams of fat.

Steakhouses

Steakhouses serve a lot of problem meals, but you can find some selections suitable for Structured Eating as well. The best bets are barbecued chicken and grilled fish. If you really want red meat, what's a healthy choice? Filet mignon or sirloin, which are both lean cuts. Since a heart-healthy diet contains only six ounces of meat, fish, poultry, and cheese a day, one option is to split a nine-ounce sirloin steak with another member of your party. Each of you then orders a salad, a side of steamed vegetables, and maybe a baked potato—about 200 calories, approximately 7 grams of fat.

For Web-based nutrition info, check the Outback Steakhouse site (www.outback.com), which explains how to order a low-fat, low-calorie meal. The Lone Star Steakhouse and Saloon site (www.lonestarsteak house.com) also provides nutrition data.

Cracker Barrel

At this chain, the pot roast is a good option for Structured Eating. A whole order is 10 ounces, so ask for half—185 calories, 3 grams of fat. Double the vegetables—approximately 125 calories, 6 grams of fat. One baked potato with a tablespoon of sour cream—slightly over 300 calories, 3 grams of fat. The total for the meal is a little less than 600 calories, about 10 grams of fat.

Subway

For a healthy sandwich, try the six-inch sub. If you order a six-inch turkey breast sub without the cheese and the mayonnaise but with lettuce, tomato, onion, green pepper, and olives, its total will be 280 calories, 4.5 grams of fat. Then there is the Veggie Delite salad with two ounces of fat-free dressing. (Keep in mind that the dressing is probably very high in sodium.) Use half of the dressing on the salad and half on your turkey breast sandwich. Order a diet soda. The total: 376 calories, 5.5 grams of fat.

Au Bon Pain

Many people think of wrap sandwiches as diet food. The problem with wraps, unfortunately, is that they're huge. The way out of this dilemma: order a healthy wrap—something with a little turkey and lots of lettuce and tomato—and then limit the amount of mayonnaise. Eat just half. These sandwiches are way too big, so pick the healthiest one and eat only half. Au Bon Pain also offers salads and soups that are low-cal, tasty, and nutritious.

Burger King

This chain used to have the highest-calorie, highest-fat sandwich, but another fast-food chain now holds that dubious honor. In any case, the Double Whopper with Cheese (1,060 calories, 69 grams of fat) is the equivalent of three whole meals here at Structure House. Add the Burger King supersized fries (600 calories, 30 grams of fat) and the large chocolate milk shake (850 calories, 27 grams of fat) for a total of 2,510 calories, 126 grams of fat. Unfortunately, even Burger King's high-fat sandwich has been outdone by Hardee's.

For a better bet for Structure at Burger King, try the Fire-grilled Chicken Caesar Salad with fat-free honey mustard—190 calories without dressing, 260 with.

Another option: Shrimp Caesar Salad with fat-free honey mustard—180 calories without the dressing, 250 with dressing added.

Wendy's

A good option here would be the Mandarin Chicken Salad without the dressing—170 calories, 3 grams of fat. A packet of crispy rice noodles would add 60 calories, 2 grams of fat. Alternatively, there's the Ultimate Grilled Chicken Sandwich with 360 calories, 7 grams of fat. Salads at Wendy's include the Spring Mix with fat-free dressing—with dressing, 260 calories; without, 180.

McDonald's

The Golden Arches offers a grilled chicken Caesar salad—220 calories, 6 grams of fat. With Newman's Own low-fat balsamic vinaigrette added, the salad clocks in at 140 calories, 3 grams of fat. A side salad is 20 calories, 0 grams of fat.

Boston Market

A healthy choice here would be the Hand-carved Rotisserie Turkey, steamed vegetable medley, and seasonal fruit salad—240 calories, 6 grams of fat. This chain has lots of good vegetable side dishes, too, such as zucchini marinara.

Panera Bread

Here's a good bet for Structured Eating: the Asian Sesame Chicken Salad with just two tablespoons of dressing—just over 300 calories, about 10 grams of fat. Another excellent choice is the low-fat vegetarian garden vegetable soup at slightly more than 90 calories, 0.5 gram of fat. Other options include the low-fat vegetarian Moroccan tomato-lentil soup—8 ounces provide 120 calories, 1.5 grams of fat—and the low-fat chicken-noodle soup—1 cup provides 90 calories, 0.5 gram of fat.

TASK 3: STRUCTURED EATING AT ETHNIC RESTAURANTS

One of the most remarkable cultural developments in this country over the past several decades has been the spread of ethnic restaurants throughout the land. Even twenty or thirty years ago, "ethnic food" in much of the United States, at least outside of the major cities, was pretty well limited to Italian, Chinese, and perhaps Mexican restaurants. "High-end" international food meant French cuisine, end of story. Now a vast range of ethnic restaurants has spread nationwide: Thai, Indian, Caribbean, Japanese, South American, Eastern European, Vietnamese, Russian, Ethiopian—you name it. The quality varies, of course, as is true everywhere, but the variety is a huge change from the past.

Ethnic restaurants, like chain establishments, can be nutritional minefields. But if you arrive knowing what to eat, you can make these varied and delightful cuisines a part of Structured Eating. As always, the trick is to know what to expect and then plan your meals with the principles of Structure in mind.

Here's an overview of several international cuisines and how to stay Structured while enjoying them.

Chinese

When Chinese restaurateurs serve their customers in this country, they don't provide the authentic Chinese food still eaten in the rural villages of

China. The traditional Chinese diet is plant-based, includes only one or two ounces of meat, fish, or poultry a day, and derives only 10 to 15 percent of its calories from fat. Most Americans wouldn't respond favorably to this diet. For this reason, the proprietors of Chinese restaurants feed us what *we* prefer: lots of animal protein and lots of fat. A typical stir-fried dish might contain three or four tablespoons of oil—300 to 400 calories' worth. (A tablespoon of oil has 120 calories.)

What does this mean about eating at Chinese restaurants? I recommend this approach: pick a dish that has lots of vegetables and little bits of meat, fish, or poultry as an accent to the dish. That's the way the Chinese really eat. Ideally, have the dish steamed, rather than stir-fried. Ask for the sauce on the side. Sauce of this sort is usually broth-based with ginger, scallions, white wine, a small amount of soy sauce or oyster sauce, and tapioca starch as a thickener. Specify no oil or fat in the sauce. Ideally, request the use of only a quarter or half teaspoon of soy sauce. Chinese food is often high in sodium—but this issue is common for many types of restaurant food. A single tablespoon of soy sauce contains 1,200 milligrams of sodium. Since the recommended intake of sodium is no more than 2,300 milligrams per day (ideally, 1,500 milligrams), it's difficult—if not impossible—to stay within this limit at restaurants, but perhaps even more so at Asian restaurants. Here's a good example of a healthy Chinese meal. Start off with hot-and-sour soup—110 calories, 4 grams of fat. Then order half a cup of steamed rice (120 calories, 0 gram of fat) with three cups of steamed vegetables (120 calories, 0 gram of fat) and three ounces of steamed shrimp (90 calories, 1.5 grams of fat). Add two tablespoons of the sauce you requested *on the side,* and you've got a total of 450 calories and 4.5 grams of fat.

Italian

Although restaurants in Italy often emphasize vegetables and provide modest portions of meat and pasta, it's easy to get Unstructured at an Italian restaurant in the United States. With garlic bread and antipasti on the table as you settle in, you can consume hundreds of calories even before you order your entrée. Fried calamari and similar appetizers are high-calorie, high-fat fare. And signature dishes like fettuccine Alfredo clock in at upward of 1,500 calories and almost 100 grams of fat.

So what's a healthy approach to Italian cuisine? For your entrée, request an appetizer-sized serving of pasta with a tomato-based sauce. Or else order a half serving of linguini with red clam sauce: 446 calories, 11.5 grams of fat. Add to that two cups of salad—vegetables with no croutons, bacon bits, or cheese: 20 calories and 0 gram of fat. The dressing? To avoid high-calorie house dressings, bring your own dressing in individual packets, or else have the waiter bring you some balsamic vinegar. If you want vegetables, order a cup of steamed veggies—40 to 50 calories, 0 gram of fat. (Keep in mind, however, that chain restaurants often prepare the steamed vegetables in individual microwavable packets that often contain some butter or margarine. So at a chain restaurant, a cup of steamed vegetables will probably provide about 50 to 60 calories and 2 to 4 grams of fat.) After the meal, order decaf espresso with no-cal sweetener. Your total for this meal: 506 calories, 11.5 grams of fat.

Mexican

If you've ever traveled to Mexico, you know that the huge open-air markets there are filled with beautiful fresh produce. The food that Mexicans prepare for themselves has a strong emphasis on vegetables—especially tomatoes, squash, spinach, other leafy vegetables, and corn—as well as an abundance of fresh fruit. The southern states of Puebla and Oaxaca, especially, are celebrated for their vibrant regional cuisines. The Gulf Coast state of Veracruz is famous for fine seafood dishes. Unfortunately, these cuisines are rarely evident at Mexican restaurants in the United States. Most U.S. Mexican restaurants tend to emphasize the high-calorie, high-fat, high-sodium ingredients more typical of Tex-Mex fare. My recommendation: *Select your Mexican restaurant with caution.*

To avoid bogging down in meals laden with lard, sour cream, cheese, and fried meats, here are some suggestions for a Structured approach to Mexican food. Order soft chicken tacos (about 200 calories, 10 to 11 grams of fat) and half a cup of Mexican rice (approximately 150 calories, about 3 to 4 grams of fat). Add two tablespoons of *picante* sauce—around

10 calories, 0 gram of fat. A garden salad with fat-free dressing (slightly under 30 calories, 0 gram of fat) and a diet soda will contribute to a total for the meal of just over 400 calories, around 12 grams of fat. Note: large tortillas tend to be very calorie-dense. Although taco salads may seem like a healthy option, they are often one of the worst items on the menu. Why? The culprit is the big fried shell.

Greek

Most of the cuisines we're discussing are much healthier in their countries of origin. This holds true for Mediterranean food, including Greek cuisine. Here again, the meals in these countries often use a much higher proportion of vegetables than U.S. Middle Eastern restaurants do, but you'd never know it from a Greek meal like *moussaka*, which includes fried eggplant, ground beef, and cheese—a very fat-intensive dish.

By contrast, here's a healthy Greek meal. Order chicken *souvlaki*, which is a kind of kebab. This dish is a Middle Eastern variant on a foolproof approach: eating simply. Broiled or grilled chicken or fish is almost always a good start. *Souvlaki* is simple fare, but it seems special because it's on a skewer and nicely spiced. This kebab comes out to 260 calories, 8 grams of fat. Add half a cup of Greek rice—80 calories, 2.5 grams of fat—and three cups of Greek salad without dressing and without feta cheese (140 calories and 3 grams of fat). If you add a half ounce of feta cheese, that's another 40 calories and 3 grams of fat. You may want to add some balsamic vinegar to the salad.

Japanese

For healthy Japanese food, sushi is the way to go. Here's a rule of thumb for sushi: most kinds of fish (with the exception of salmon) have about 32 calories per ounce. Rice, too, has about 32 calories an ounce. The bottom line: sushi will have about 32 calories per ounce regardless of the proportion of fish to rice. Given the benefits of eating fish plus the low-fat preparation of Japanese rice, sushi is always a good choice. Six pieces of raw tuna sushi shaped onto small beds of rice—that's 228 calories, 0 gram of fat. You could order some *edamame* (boiled soybeans) to go with it. A good side dish might be green seaweed salad, which is a crinkly, tasty vegetable often prepared with a light, sweetened vinegar dressing or a dash of sesame oil.

Japanese food is generally a healthy cuisine, but be aware of the high fat content of some broiled dishes, such as chicken or beef teriyaki, and the even higher fat content of fried *yakitori* and *tempura* dishes. Also, Asian cuisines in general tend to be high in sodium. (Then again, almost *all* restaurant foods are high in sodium.)

Indian

Indian food presents some tough dilemmas. The many cuisines of India are delicious, but they can be problematic because the cooks use *ghee*, or clarified butter, a very highly saturated fat that raises blood cholesterol levels more than any other kind. To complicate matters, the highest-fat, highest-calorie dishes are often vegetarian. Consider *palak paneer*, a spinach dish that contains large quantities of whole-milk cheese. The Indian bread called *nan* also contains a lot of *ghee*. Basmati rice, too, is always prepared with *ghee*.

The healthy Indian meal I'll describe was prepared by an intern who worked at Structure House while finishing her M.S. degree in nutrition at the University of North Carolina. Originally from India, she had come to this country to finish her education. Here's the meal. First, *chapatis*—an Indian whole-wheat bread. One piece of *chapati* or plain *roti* (another kind of Indian bread) has 145 calories and 5 grams of fat. For a main course, the best choice is shrimp biryani—286 calories, 8 grams of fat. Then three tablespoons of vegetable *raita*, a cucumber-tomato-onion chutney—24 calories, 0 gram of fat. Add sliced mango (107 calories, 0 gram of fat) for a total of 562 calories, 13 grams of fat.

"To Your Health"

In many cultures, the toast or blessing before a meal offers good health to everyone present. This is the ideal goal as we eat: health and long life. It's certainly an attainable goal, too, if you select your foods thoughtfully.

Here's what I'll tell you about restaurant eating: You don't have to go into social isolation. You don't have to limit yourself to bland foods. You can stay Structured in almost any cuisine you fancy. Whether you prefer good ol' American cooking or something more exotic, you have *many* options for Structured Eating.

Some final suggestions for staying Structured in restaurants:

- Certain restaurants are famous for huge portions, so avoid them if at all possible.
- All-you-can-eat buffets automatically present major problems for Structured Eating, so avoid them, too.
- Going out with "overeating buddies" is a setup for trouble.
- When you can't preplan, order simple food like grilled fish or grilled chicken plus a baked potato and a salad.
- Unless you're an expert, it's very difficult (if not impossible) to control sodium intake at a restaurant. If you have high blood pressure, you don't really want to eat at restaurants very often. Consider heart-healthy or low-salt selections if they're on the menu.
- Be clear with people at the restaurant regarding what you need. If that means low-sodium, press the point. If you want low-fat, press the point. Then, if the waiter brings you a meal that's clearly too salty or too rich, you won't feel guilty when you send it back. Do your homework well in advance; call ahead to ask questions; and be specific but polite when you're ordering.

TASK 4: MEET THE CHALLENGES OF STRUCTURED EATING WHILE TRAVELING

When starting your journey with Structured Eating, dining away from the comfort of home can be a challenge. These challenges are especially numerous when you're traveling beyond your own area. Just some of the issues to consider when staying Structured include destination, mode of travel, accommodations, and uncertainty about whether nutritious food will be available. But don't worry. You can stay Structured during your travels from start to finish. One of the truly great things about the Structure House approach is that it's totally portable. Wherever you go, it's right there in your new skills and attitudes.

First, let's ask some questions to clarify the issues; then I'll share some tips to make Structured Eating manageable "on the road."

Does spontaneous travel have a place in a Structured world?

Remember: Structured Eating means consuming three meals a day that are planned, nutritious, and consistent with your calorie goal. Therefore, deciding on the time, place, and content of your meals will be essential. Is this planning possible if you don't know in advance where you are going, how you will be getting there, or where you will be staying? Maybe—but it's not likely. For this reason, the best starting point for Structured Eating during trips is to create a travel itinerary. This itinerary should include the following information:

- Your destination
- Your mode of travel
- Your housing plans
- Your meal choices

Can you stay Structured during international travel?

Where you go is truly a personal choice. However, your destination may affect the relative ease or difficulty of staying Structured. When traveling in the United States, for instance, you can be fairly confident that wherever you go you will find familiar foods. You can also be confident of your ability to communicate with other people, including vendors, restaurant personnel, and hotel staffs. This may not be true, however, for international travel, where other languages, ingredients, and cooking styles will complicate your tasks.

If you will be traveling internationally, you may find preplanning meals more difficult, and you'll probably need to devote some time and effort to investigating the food culture of your chosen destination. Ideally, familiarize yourself with commonly available types of foods and their nutritional content. Some options:

- **Familiarize yourself with common cooking methods and local beliefs or customs about food preparation.** One option: Visit a bookstore and look through the cookbook section. Even a cursory overview of books specific to the cuisine you'll be eating will give you lots of ideas about which foods are available and how they're prepared. Trolling the Web for information is another option.

- **Learn at least some of the host country's language.** Fluency isn't necessary, but learning to recognize and say key words and phrases for food items, cooking methods, and restaurant etiquette will make staying Structured far easier while traveling. If necessary, get help translating food-related terms and sentences you'll need, such as "steamed," "broiled," "low-salt," "without the sauce," and so forth.

- **If you live in a college town, consider contacting foreign students from the country you plan to visit.** Ask them questions about their country and its cuisine. What ingredients are typical? What dishes might lend themselves to Structured Eating? Can these students recommend specific restaurants? Many will be eager to talk about their own culture with interested Americans.

- **Consider picking up a travel guide that includes key phrases for ordering at a restaurant in the country you'll be visiting.** Most phrasebooks (such as those published by Berlitz, Lonely Planet, and other companies) include words and sentences that will simplify this task. One specific example: *The Berlitz European Menu Reader.*

How will you get there?

Of the four most common modes of travel—car, plane, boat, and train—each presents its own advantages and disadvantages as you try to stay Structured.

Car

When planning your travel itinerary, take time to plan your route. If possible, attempt to Structure, prepare, and pack your own meals for the trip. Consider keeping a restaurant resource guide such as *Restaurant Confi-*

dential in your glove compartment, which will help you find the nutrition information for menu items available at stops along your route. One option: Abandon the Interstate! Or at least take part of your trip on the grid of "blue highways" that will give you a far better picture of the land and the people who live there. The food may be better, too. Instead of stopping at the same old chain restaurants, you will have a chance to discover some local favorites.

Plane

Virtually all major airlines offer special meals, including low-calorie, low-sodium, kosher, and vegetarian. However, you need to make your request well in advance. Consider placing your request at the time you book your ticket to ensure that you receive the appropriate meal. It's no secret that in recent years, airlines have tried to cut costs by limiting meal and beverage service on most flights. If your flight doesn't include meal service, or if you face a long layover, you may need to consider eating at the airport.

The good news: Most airports now offer a variety of restaurants and counter services for meals. The bad news: The food available is often high-calorie, high-fat, high-sodium fare. I recommend that you investigate the airport prior to arriving there to determine where you'll be eating and what sorts of meals will be available. One way to accomplish this goal: use a Web site such as AirNav.com. By looking for restaurants that provide nutrition information within the facility, you may find staying Structured easier than you thought. If you find that the restaurants or meals available at the airport don't offer appropriate choices, however, consider prepacking your meal.

It's true that many carriers have downsized in-flight food almost to the vanishing point. Some haven't, though. (For example, Continental continues to offer meal service on many flights.) If you're on such a flight, take a tip from savvy travelers: request specialized meals from the airline. The more unusual your needs, the more individualized the attention you'll receive. One person I know orders diabetic vegetarian kosher dinners—even though she isn't diabetic, vegetarian, or Jewish! Why? Because the meal is so out of the ordinary that it's bound to get special attention. She reports that the food has been excellent and consistent with Structured Eating.

Boat

We've all heard tales about cruise liners. Bountiful buffets and extravagant meals are available at every turn, and people speak of gaining ten pounds or more on just a long weekend cruise. It sounds more like a structureless nightmare than a great vacation.

My suggestion: explore what several cruise lines have to offer before you book your ticket. Try to locate a cruise that offers more formal dining arrangement, such as sit-down meals with a full-service waitstaff. This will allow for greater opportunities to preplan more accurately and modify your meals as needed. Many cruise lines offer healthy dining programs as well, so do some research before you make your reservation. Once you're on board, take advantage of all of the fresh fruits and vegetables, but steer clear of the midnight buffet! Also, don't forget that cruise lines offer a variety of daily activities to keep you physically active—gyms, swimming, aerobics, dancing, and many others. One last suggestion: Avoid all the cruise lines that boast 24/7 food. The last thing you want is to spend a week on what's essentially a floating all-you-can-eat joint.

Train

Within the United States, the major rail line is Amtrak. Not all Amtrak routes offer meal service; for those that do, however, seventy-two-hour advance notice may give you the option of accommodating certain dietary needs, including kosher and vegetarian meals, as well as requesting reduced-sodium or reduced-cholesterol selections.

Train travel is popular in European countries. A Eurailpass will get you onto trains on a network of railroads that provides service to eighteen European countries. While purchasing a Eurailpass or regular tickets will give you the freedom to move quickly from one country to another, it doesn't guarantee that services will be consistent. Services such as first-class access or meal and beverage service vary from country to country. It's best to contact the rail service provider within your country of travel for more details on the amenities provided (this can often be done on the Internet). Once again, consider taking a healthy meal with you.

Where will you stay?

Following decisions about transportation, the next issue you face is lodging.

Hotels and Motels

When you make your reservations, consider staying in a facility that offers a kitchen or kitchenette—a great opportunity for creating your own Structured meals. If a kitchenette isn't available, however, discuss room service selections and the proximity of local markets and restaurants with the hotel concierge. Contact those businesses and investigate what food choices are available.

Many hotels are now offering a greater abundance of healthy foods on their menus. Check in advance to determine when room service is available; you don't want to arrive hungry and have to resort to the vending machines. In addition, do some research on restaurants in the area by using Web sites such as Citysearch (www.citysearch.com) or Zagat Survey (www.zagat.com) to see which restaurants will best meet your needs.

Bed-and-Breakfasts

Most B&Bs offer homemade breakfasts, and some offer other meals as well. When making your reservation, you'll have the perfect opportunity to interview the owner or manager—who may, in fact, be the chef as well. Discuss what meals will be served and what menu items will be offered, as well as an overview of the ingredients that will be used and the cooking methods employed. Ask if the establishment will be willing to accommodate special requests.

Keep in mind that traditionally, B&Bs serve breakfast but no other meals. A limited number have restaurants on site or affiliated with the lodging. If the B&B you'll visit is among the majority that serve only breakfast, ask the innkeeper about the possibility of using the kitchen facilities yourself to prepare your own lunch or dinner.

Private Rental Home or Apartment

This arrangement has the advantage of providing a kitchen on site. In addition, the owners will have information available about local food stores and restaurants. Why complicate your life? Stay in, prepare your own preplanned meals, and rest easy.

An Adventure, Not a Problem

By definition, travel means that you leave what's familiar and seek what's less familiar. Change comes with the turf. Is that kind of change a challenge? Of course! But the challenges of travel—experiencing new places, meeting new people, and doing new activities—are part of what prompts so many people to leave the comforts of home behind and seek new horizons. Traveling means that you accept the necessity of change. But as is often true in other situations, the change inherent in travel is an adventure, not a problem.

Here are some final suggestions to make this adventure easier and more enjoyable.

Seek Help in Planning

What we've discussed in this chapter covers a lot of terrain ("terrain" in more ways than one). If you feel overwhelmed by the travel-planning tasks involved, don't hesitate to seek advice. A good travel agent can smooth the path before you. Increasingly, the travel industry will take customers' dietary and nutritional needs into account as part of the planning process. But ultimately *you* are the person who calls the shots. Take responsibility for your diet and health issues. Play the most active role possible regarding food issues: which restaurants to visit, when to eat, and so forth. Take control of your life.

Use Your Knowledge of the Structure House Program

While planning your travel itinerary, consider what obstacles you may encounter. Take time to review this book before you set out on your trip, and consider how the concepts outlined can help you overcome any obstacles as you travel.

Make a Backup Plan for Your Meals

What happens if your plans for Structured Eating fall through during your trip? That's always a possibility. Travel is nothing if not uncertain. Perhaps your flight is delayed, so you reach your hotel after the restaurant has closed. Or the great café a friend recommended turns out to have gone belly-up. Or else there's a holiday in progress when you arrive in your host country and restaurants and food stores alike are closed. Under these and other circumstances, how do you find nutritious food that meets your dietary needs?

There's no easy response to this question, but here are some suggestions for nutritional "emergencies":

- Many cities and towns overseas—especially in Europe—have cafés with extended service hours in the municipal train stations. Some of the larger stations even have their own grocery stores.

- Fresh produce is widely available almost anywhere you're likely to travel. If you can't find restaurants whose fare appeals to you, tide yourself over by purchasing fruits and vegetables.

- Don't expect to be perfect. There will be times when you can't stay Structured. If you arrive late in an unfamiliar town, find only one restaurant open, and end up eating a meal that doesn't fit your plans, it's not the end of the world. Don't berate yourself. Don't regard yourself as having "failed." Just consider the situation a result of stressful circumstances, move on, and get back to Structure the next day.

Finally, I want to tell you that for many years, I've heard some people tell me that "you just can't stay Structured while traveling." They say it can't be done—and that's that. Well, I think this is an unfortunate point of view. I said this earlier, but I want to say it again: *You can Structure any situation.* No matter where you are or what you're doing, Structure is "in there" somewhere. You can find it. You can create it. You just have to consider the possibilities, experiment, and see what works.

The task isn't insurmountable. Whether you're visiting a nearby town, driving across the United States, vacationing in Paris, attending a convention in Chicago, or taking a Caribbean cruise, you can create Structure. How? By breaking the trip into small steps. Ask yourself, "Where will I be for meal 1?," "Where will I be for meal 2?," and so on. Then plan what you'll be doing.

Like travel itself, you don't take the whole journey all at once. *Step by step is how you get there.*

CHAPTER 9

Maintain the Structured Mind-set: More Tools for the Structure House Toolbox

"You can't do it alone. You have to have a support system—whether that support system is e-mail, a therapist, a friend who's willing to listen, a support group of overeaters, or a combination of all of the above. Don't isolate yourself to just one thing."

—Sallie

"You're learning a skill that you've never had before in your life. But to gain that skill, you have to practice, practice, practice."

—Arthur

"Find friends who understand and support you. I always encourage people to find other people in the same situation and talk about it."

—Aaron

Imagine that you're a carpenter. You grab your toolbox and head for work to build a house. On reaching the construction site, you notice that the toolbox seems lighter than usual, and you discover on raising the lid that the only tool inside the box is a hammer. This is an unnerving discovery! You sure hope your work today will be limited to pounding nails! But the odds are that you'll probably also have to saw some boards, plane some doors, and drill some holes. How are you going to perform these tasks with nothing but a hammer? You'll surely run into some problems—and you'll probably never finish the house.

For all of us, our personalities are our inner toolboxes. The tools inside the box are our fixing skills. When we face a stressful situation or a problem, we reach into this toolbox for "tools"—some sort of resource for fixing what we face. The more tools we have at hand, the greater our ability to fix life effectively.

What are the tools in your toolbox? Perhaps you have a great variety of tools available. Unfortunately, it's also possible that your toolbox resembles that of the carpenter I described above. Perhaps you have only one tool available for responding to all your problems and challenges. If that one response to problems and challenges is eating, then you probably:

- Use food as a companion when you're lonely
- Use food as a tranquilizer when you're anxious
- Use food as a safety valve when you're angry
- Use food as entertainment when you're bored
- Use food as a form of tension release when you're stressed

I could go on and on.

We have a lot of participants at Structure House who arrive here with a one-tool toolbox. They'll say, "I eat when I'm lonely, I eat when I'm social, I eat when I'm busy, and I eat when I'm bored. I eat to ease pain when my body aches, and I eat to celebrate when my body feels good." Someone who describes his or her responses in these words is using food as the primary (or only) response to a diverse and complex set of situations. This is a person whose toolbox is incomplete.

Why is this approach a problem? It's a problem because, at least in the long run, it backfires. What starts as a solution becomes a bigger and bigger problem in its own right. Your almost empty toolbox limits what you can fix—and, in fact, it creates more difficulties than you can solve. You gain weight, damage your health, lose your mobility, diminish your social life, reduce your self-esteem, and limit your level of activity. As these negative side effects accumulate, you habitually reward and comfort yourself with the only thing that your toolbox provides: food.

How can you change this situation? Add tools to your toolbox. Create a toolbox that's more complete and more adaptable than what you're using now. Acquire tools that will allow you to create the most numerous and effective responses to what you face in life.

What are these "tools"? They are skills for long-term weight control, lifestyle change, and stress management. Over time, you can increase the number of tools—fixing skills—in your toolbox. *As with every other aspect of the Structure House approach, adding and using these tools is a long-term, lifelong process, not a quick fix.*

TOOL 1: MONITOR AND MANAGE CHANGE

If you've used fad diets in the past, you've probably been accustomed to quick-fix approaches that promise dramatic results in a very short time. Have these promises been fulfilled? What most people experience on a fad diet is that they lose some weight initially, then bounce back to their original weight—or put on even more pounds than before. By contrast, the Structure House approach values steady, long-term change. This approach offers greater benefits than fad diets do, but it also presents the challenge of taking a long view.

Let's start by asking two important questions:

- How do you know how you're changing?
- How do you monitor change?

To begin to answer the first question, let's review the journey so far by means of a checklist that many Structure House participants have found useful.

Reviewing Change

Here are some issues that may have changed for you.

- Put a check mark beside each issue that you know has changed.
- Put a question mark beside each issue that you aren't sure about.

Remember: there are no "right" or "wrong" answers—just your personal responses. This exercise serves simply to assess your situation as you undertake the journey toward change.

Old Attitude or Assumption

____ 1. I weigh too much because of my metabolism.

____ 2. I have certain health problems that stop me from losing and controlling my weight.

____ 3. I am confused about weight loss, metabolism of fat, and the sodium in my body.

____ 4. I feel I do not eat enough to be so overweight.

____ 5. I feel the scale is important and hope to see weight loss every day.

____ 6. I have been told many things about diets and am confused.

____ 7. I am not aware of portion sizes and calorie amounts.

____ 8. Family members don't have to be cooperative. I have to do this myself.

New Attitude or Assumption

____ 1. I weigh too much because I eat too much.

____ 2. I am healthy, and any health problems I have will resolve after weight loss. I can now concentrate on the changes I must make.

____ 3. I understand now about weight loss, metabolism of fat, and the sodium in my body.

____ 4. I am now aware of how much I eat.

____ 5. I realize that my behavior is more important and the scale is not indicative of behavior; I don't expect daily weight loss.

____ 6. I am now aware of proper nutrition and what a balanced diet is.

____ 7. I am now aware of portions and calorie amounts.

____ 8. I must have my family's cooperation if I am to succeed.

____ 9. Whoever prepares the meal doesn't have to help me; I don't have to eat it.

____10. I never plan my meals, weigh myself every day, or keep track of what I'm doing.

____ 9. I need the help of whomever prepares the meals.

____10. I realize that I must Structure my meals, weigh myself every day, and keep a diary if I'm going to know what to do and how I am doing.

Now that you can see the ways in which you've changed—and perhaps the ways in which you haven't—it's important to make some decisions. How are you going to make the changes that will benefit you? Do you even know what changes you want to make? Here are some suggestions for fostering change:

- Write out the changes you want to make.
- Write out how you want these changes to take place.
- If you know how you want things in your life to be different, write out the changes you'd like to have happen.
- Take these steps occasionally to determine what changes to make.

Keep in mind that as far as change is concerned, there are three likely scenarios:

- You can make things happen.
- You can let things happen to you.
- Or you can wonder what happened (or why it didn't happen).

Which of these scenarios is what you want for yourself?

As you think over these issues, I want you to keep the following suggestions in mind:

- **Focus on food, not weight.** You have more control over what and how you eat, less control over what the dial on the scale shows you on any specific day.

- **Expect plateaus and maintenance periods.** Weight loss won't be steady or continuous. Many people lose weight more quickly at the start of a weight loss program, then more gradually.

- **Consider tracking BMI instead of pounds.** BMI takes height into consideration and is a better indication of your "danger zone."

- **Consider also tracking other changes:** your measurements, your clothing sizes, your overall flexibility, and your cardiovascular ability.

- **Give lots of attention to exercise,** which can improve your fitness regardless of weight. (We discuss exercise in detail in Chapter 7.)

- **Avoid exaggerating the importance and benefits of numerical weight.** Yes, you're trying to lose weight, but there are a lot of issues to consider beyond just the number the needle is pointing to.

- **Consider that there may be reasons why an "ideal weight" you're striving for is unattainable.** Pay attention to other criteria for improvement rather than weight alone.

- **Try to separate your weight from your self-esteem.** You are far more interesting, complex, and capable than anything that can be expressed as a number on a scale!

People sometimes ask me if they can make changes fast—changes to their weight, their lifestyle, or both. They seem concerned that with Structured Eating as the core principle, the transitions will happen too slowly. I feel sympathetic to their eagerness, but haste isn't the best approach. Unlike the situation with dependence on drugs and alcohol, where the treatment of choice is to go "cold turkey," you can't take that approach with a dependence on food. You have to learn to live with food and adjust your habits over a period of time. Staying Structured is the best method for learning to live with food, adjusting to new ways of thinking about food, improving your health, and fostering change in how you live.

The tools in your toolbox are the coping skills you acquire and practice as you live your life. Monitoring and mastering change, using Structured Eating as a long-term strategy for change, and managing stress are among the most powerful and adaptable tools available for dealing with the challenges you face. These tools give you effective ways for dealing with life on a day-to-day basis, and they also help you to avoid Unstructured Eating in response to the antecedents, or "eating triggers," of habit, boredom, and stress.

TOOL 2: LEARN FROM SUCCESSFUL WEIGHT LOSERS

If you're interested in mastering a complex skill, one of the best ways to "learn the ropes" is to understand how practitioners of the same skill have attained success. This approach holds true whether the skill in question involves playing cards, sailing boats, tending a garden, repairing cars, or raising children. It's also true about losing weight. Many people are successful at losing weight and solving weight-related health problems. Who are these people, and what can we learn from their efforts to lose weight? Fortunately, you don't have to do any research to find them. A number of interesting, useful studies are already under way—some of them tracking the participants over many years—and the information from these studies is readily available. This research provides a useful tool for your toolbox: learning from successful weight losers.

Probably the best research under way is an ongoing study by the National Weight Control Registry. This study focuses on a population of 4,000 to 5,000 men and women who are being tracked over the long term to monitor their consistent success in losing weight and maintaining their weight loss. Headed by a psychologist named Rena Wing at Brown University, the National Weight Control Registry research observes people who are losing weight within organized programs, as well as some people who are losing weight on their own. The researchers' goal is to understand better the common denominators of success among people who have been able to lose weight effectively.[1]

Here's a summary of what this research has revealed so far, including questions about the participants and the patterns of how these men and women are achieving their success in weight loss and weight maintenance:

Minimum Qualifications for the Registry

The participants need to have lost at least thirty pounds and kept it off at least one year. The average person in the registry has lost fifty to sixty pounds and has kept it off for five years.

Were the people in the registry overweight as children?

Forty-six percent became overweight before age 12, and another 25 percent became overweight by age 19.

Did the people in the registry have overweight parents?

Seventy-three percent of the people in the registry had at least one overweight parent.

Had these people previously tried to lose weight?

Yes, 91 percent had unsuccessfully tried to lose weight and keep it off in the past.

How was their strategy different during this attempt?

Eighty-one percent exercised more than during previous attempts, and 63 percent employed a stricter dietary approach.

How did they lose weight?

Almost all of the participants (89 percent) modified both diet and physical activity in order to lose weight and keep it off.

How did their eating change?

Ninety-two percent limited the quantities of certain types of food, 49 percent limited the quantities of food eaten, 38 percent limited calories from fat, and 35 percent counted calories. Less than 1 percent ate high-protein, low-carbohydrate diets. The average fat intake was 24 percent of total calories.

How much exercise did they do to maintain their weight loss?

These participants averaged 2,700 calories of exercise per week. This is equivalent to walking four miles or one hour each day.

How often did they dine out?

They ate less than one meal per week in fast-food restaurants and only two meals per week in non-fast-food restaurants.

How did the quality of their lives change after successfully keeping off their lost weight?

At least 85 percent reported improvements in general quality of life, level of energy, physical mobility, general mood, self-confidence, and physical health.

Did they feel it was more difficult to lose or maintain their lost weight?

Most (42 percent) thought weight loss was more difficult. Only 25 percent felt weight maintenance was more difficult.

Given what these National Weight Control Registry participants describe—and given what other successful weight losers have to say about their experiences in other studies—let's consider what can you learn from them and apply to your own situation.

What Is "Success"?

First, let's clarify what we're discussing. When we talk about "successful weight losers," what do we mean by "success"? Is it simply a matter of how many pounds they've lost? Is it how long they've kept off the pounds? Or does success include other criteria? In fact, there's no set definition of "success" in the field of weight loss; the interpretation of this term varies from study to study.

Some years ago, an article in a professional journal within the obesity field ventured an opinion that professionals in this field have gotten stuck in a narrow perception of success. There's been a tendency to interpret success solely by a quantitative measure: the number of pounds lost. However, it's increasingly evident that we need to perceive success in broader terms. If you consider only the number of pounds lost, you ignore a lot of important factors. Not long ago, for instance, I observed a group of Structure House participants applaud another participant because, for the first time in this woman's stay, she had managed to walk up the stairs rather than taking the elevator from the first floor to the second. A huge event had taken place in her life. You would miss the significance of that event if you looked only at the number of pounds this participant had lost. You would also miss health improvements in her and other people—improvements in blood pressure, cholesterol level, blood sugar level, joint health, and other factors. You would miss improvements in use of medications. You would miss improvements in fitness levels and changes in body measurements, clothing sizes, moods, confidence, and self-esteem.

In short, "success" is multidimensional, not just a number on the scale or even a sequence of numbers on a weight chart. And successful weight losers often emphasize factors that go far beyond these numbers.

Suggestions from Successful Weight Losers

Following are some of the issues that successful weight losers raise as instrumental in their efforts.

Find Social Support

A common theme in discussions of successful weight loss is the benefit of finding support among other people. There are many ways for you to build in more support for yourself as you strive for long-term weight loss. Some people join Overeaters Anonymous (OA) and find that group comfortable and useful. Others join Weight Watchers, which provides a community of like-minded people. Still others hire a personal trainer, a nutritionist, or a psychotherapist. All of these are legitimate forms of support. What will you do to boost your support system?

A later section of this chapter will offer some specific suggestions.

Self-Monitor

According to the National Weight Control Registry, self-monitoring is one of the most important elements of what successful people do in working toward their goals. Self-monitoring techniques are ways of making a commitment to being honest with yourself as you pursue weight loss and improved health. There's an understandable tendency to sweep some issues under the rug. For this reason, making a commitment to self-monitoring is a fundamental foundation for success. How should you proceed?

In the Structure House approach, the Structure House Diary is the primary tool for self-monitoring. When you use the diary, you're tracking everything you eat. You're looking at your antecedents. You're looking at the connections among your lifestyle, the situations you face, and how you're dealing with food. You're weighing yourself and tracking your weight as it changes. The Structure House Diary is a powerful but flexible tool for self-monitoring.

Some people have reservations about using the diary. One reason is that it's small—there's not much space there, and you have to write in it by hand. If that's an issue, I'd say don't use our diary—try something that provides a larger format and more space. Experiment with other kinds of notebooks. You can even create a digital document on your computer. In one way or another, though, do the essentials of planning your meals and activities, noting what you eat and how your day takes shape, and tracking your antecedents to Unstructured Eating. There are all sorts of ways to monitor these data.

Accumulate Changes Incrementally

An interesting long-term study looked at people who had lost at least 20 percent of their body weight and kept the weight off for a minimum of two years.[2] The researchers invited a group of the study's subjects to get together and explain their mind-set—what they'd done and how they'd been effective. As a result of the ensuing interviews, the researchers reached what could be considered a startling conclusion: most of these people didn't think of themselves as "dieters" or regard their weight loss efforts as "going on a diet." You might think that if people lost weight and kept it off, they'd surely say, "I was on a diet." But that wasn't the case with this population. Instead, these people felt that they were simply living their lives in healthier ways. Weight loss was a natural result of the healthy behaviors that they were putting into practice incrementally. As a result of this study, you could say that it's effective to focus *more* on your behavior and *less* on the scale. Your weight will come off gradually as you engage in these healthier behaviors.

The subjects also provided a picture that didn't reveal change as *dramatic transformation* so much as *a gradual accumulation of changes*. We could imagine that, first, they'd concentrate on one behavior; then, over time, as they carried that one behavior forward, they'd add another changed behavior. They'd carry those two changes forward, then add one or two more. The implications are clear: Don't try to make all changes at once. Rather, concentrate on something specific, such as staying within your calorie count. Then you will realize what makes up those calories. Then you will start to eat less fat in your diet. Then you will add some physical activity—maybe a cardiovascular workout or strength training. Then you will add flexibility training to the cardio and the strength training. Then, as you realize you're getting in better shape, you'll start to ride your bike again, which provides you with some exercise in a way that's more fun. Little by little, you add elements. Take baby steps.

Be Flexible and Positive About Change

If they had been asked, the subjects in the study might say that they weren't perfect in following their weight loss programs. They had good days and bad days. When they had a bad day, the "setbacks" actually led to an appreciation of all the little signs of progress up to that point—signs that created a further sense of motivation to stick to the program. The implication: It pays to think positive. Ideally, you should keep some sort of log of all the changes you've made over time. Losing weight is one of those changes, but there are many, many others. You may tend to take these changes for granted if you don't make a point of keeping them in mind. I'd even suggest that you put them in writing, and, as time passes, keep adding to the list. Slowly but surely, you'll be creating a catalog of all the specific but significant changes you've accumulated. Then when you have a bad day—and everyone has them—you won't berate yourself for one small "failure." Your list of changes will help to motivate you to become Structured again.

Know What to Do When You Get Unstructured

Getting Unstructured is inevitable. It happens to everyone, and it's something you need to expect and accept as part of the process. Even if you expect and accept its inevitability, however, becoming Unstructured tends to be upsetting. You may be anxious because you may feel that even one "slip" will leave you out of control. You may feel guilty or angry toward yourself. When this happens, how should you respond?

First, stay calm! Deep breathing and other relaxation techniques may be helpful. (See the further discussion of these topics later in this chapter.) Then ask yourself what has happened. Part of the Structure House program is to explore and understand these situations. Ask yourself these questions:

- What made me vulnerable to Unstructured Eating at that particular moment?
- What were my antecedents?
- What was I feeling?
- What did I need *other* than food that prompted me to eat instead?
- Since food can be a metaphor for something else—something I need—what effect was I seeking by acting out with the food?
- What effect was I after? Was I trying to calm myself? Soothe myself? Was there some other way that I could have produced that effect?
- Can I apply what I've learned about this situation the next time I experience this antecedent?

Accept getting Unstructured as an opportunity to look more carefully at your relationship with food. If at all possible, also see it as an opportunity to take positive action—action that will help you restore a feeling of control. Sometimes the positive action is to throw out the rest of the food you were eating when you got Unstructured. Sometimes the action is realizing that you haven't made a plan to Structure your next meal, so now you'll go ahead and make a plan. Sometimes the action is taking a walk to get a boost or calling a friend for emotional support rather than resorting to more Unstructured Eating. There's always something positive you can do that will help you feel that you're restoring some control.

Remotivate Yourself

In the National Weight Control Registry research I've mentioned, participants in the study made it clear that they sometimes need to remotivate themselves to get back in sync with their programs. Perhaps you've faced the same situation. Getting Unstructured can create a motivational crisis. You may start feeling so frustrated and annoyed that you'll say, "Oh, what's the use? Why bother with all this stuff? I'll just throw it all away." These responses are normal and understandable. Rather than berating yourself for "failing," however, I urge you to see the failure as an opportunity for renewing your motivation—as an opportunity to learn. How? You have a number of options available.

One is to reread your "Dear Me" letter. This letter is an easy, accessible means of remotivating yourself. It shows you the cost, the price, the pain, and the misery you've experienced in the past. It's a clear reminder of why you're pushing hard for change—and a reminder, too, of what you may experience again if you "throw it all away." You want to move away from the hardships you've experienced. You want to enjoy the long term, not just the short term. *This* is why you're working hard to change.

Another approach is to look ahead and envision what will put staying Structured at risk. Successful weight losers ask themselves, "How am I going to handle the restaurant tomorrow night?" or "How will I cope with that social occasion at my friend's house?" If you can ask yourself these sorts of questions, you'll do better than if you don't. You're anticipating situations. You're making plans that address the challenges you've anticipated. This is an attitude that appears to produce a greater level of success.

Where will your Structure be at risk? The answer to that question will vary from person to person. An extreme example was the Structure House participant who decided that for one year, he would eat all his meals at restaurants. Why? Because for him, the high-risk situation was coping with food issues in his house. His response to this challenge led to an unusual game plan, but it worked for him! Other people would have responded with precisely the opposite approach: to do more hands-on food preparation at home and less eating in restaurants.

Here again it's best to take a gradual approach. There's evidence that people who lose weight more slowly are more likely to keep that weight off in the long run. Your approach should be "What will my life be like in three to five years?" rather than "What am I going to weigh in three to five months?" Fad programs that are designed to take weight off fast don't help much over the long term. My advice: be flexible, be patient, and constantly remotivate yourself.

Exercise

Studies of successful weight losers emphasize the importance of exercise. People tell me that it is the "glue" that keeps their program together. As we discussed in Chapter 7, exercise is one of the components of successful weight loss—ideally, a program that includes cardiovascular, strength, and flexibility training to provide a good, balanced program.

How is exercise going to fit into your life? There's evidence that early-morning exercisers are the most likely to keep up their exercise program, but that arrangement doesn't work for everybody. Consider what type of exercise you're willing to do. Do you like classes? Are you more of a solo exerciser? Would you find motivation in being part of a group, or would you prefer working with a trainer or an exercise buddy? Just think about who you are, what your preferences are, and what will work the best for you. Then commit to that kind of program. Abundant evidence suggests that your efforts will pay off.

TOOL 3: GET SUPPORT

Weight loss and lifestyle change are more challenging if you pursue them on your own. We run Structure House as a residential program precisely because the group setting offers so much support to participants. Because the book you're holding obviously isn't a group experience, I urge you to find support of *some* sort as you undertake your journey toward change. Many aspects of the process I'm describing throughout this book will be easier, more productive, and more enjoyable if you can benefit from giving support to and receiving support from other people.

The support closest at hand may be your own family. At Structure

House, we find that many relatives are eager to help a family member who's struggling with weight and health issues—but they just aren't sure what to do. You may find that as you explain the Structure House program to your immediate family, you can enlist their help in what you've undertaken. At the same time, you may have to emphasize how important the program is to you and how much you need other members' cooperation as you work to change your own lifestyle.

An alternative source of support for many people is participation in some kind of group program. Many such programs are available in American cities, and they are also increasingly available in towns and even some rural areas. Group programs provide a setting where you can discuss weight-related issues, hear about other people's experiences, and gain support for your own efforts. In addition, spending time with people who face the same issues can be tremendously helpful because of mutual support this situation can offer; when you get a desire to eat, you can call up someone and say, "I don't know what's going on. Help me figure this out." Or you can say, "My boss really frustrated me today. I'm so upset. I don't want to eat because of this. What do I do?" Ideally, your buddy will say something like "Hey, I've been there, too. Here's what I've done in situations like that." You learn from each other. You get each other through it. You're not out there on your own. A good group can provide you with both emotional support and practical expertise.

Where can you find such groups? There's no guarantee that you'll locate exactly what you want right in your area, but weight loss support groups are increasingly common throughout the United States. Here are some types of organizations that often sponsor them:

- Psychotherapy practices
- Hospitals
- Universities, colleges, and community colleges
- Churches and synagogues
- Nondenominational religious groups (such as Weigh Down and Celebrate Recovery, both Christian-oriented groups)

TOOL 4: PRACTICE RELAXATION OR MEDITATION TECHNIQUES

A wide variety of other techniques can ease tension, help you relax, and even foster insights during the process of losing weight and changing your life through the Structure House approach. Some of these methods have been perfected throughout the ages; others are more recent innovations. All can help you reach your goals for staying Structured. Try them out and see which ones you find most helpful.

Before describing these techniques, however, I'd like you to do this brief exercise.

Relaxation Self-Assessment Test

Gauge your need for relaxation techniques by answering each of the following questions with one of these responses:

A. Yes, frequently
B. Yes, sometimes
C. Occasionally
D. No, not very often
E. No, never

Have you ever suffered from, or are you currently suffering from:

_____ Insomnia (the inability to fall asleep at night)

_____ Breakthrough insomnia (awakening in the middle of the night with trouble getting back to sleep)

_____ Headaches that begin at the back of your neck and slowly work up over the scalp

_____ Headaches with a throbbing pain on one side of your head

_____ Upset stomach (including constipation, cramps, diarrhea, feelings of nausea, or sharp pains)

_____ Hypertension (high blood pressure) or angina (chest pains from heart trouble)

_____ Fatigue without physical exertion

_____ Lack of concentration or the inability to focus on what you are doing

_____ Anxiety, tension, and feeling upset without apparent reason

_____ Anxiety, tension, and feeling upset after you think you should have recovered from an upsetting episode

_____ Feeling depressed or sad

If you answered "A" even once, or if you answered "B" more than three times, I strongly urge you to consider using one or more of the relaxation techniques I'll describe to you now.

Relaxation—Not Just Time at the Beach

We all tend to assume that relaxation means getting away: going on vacation, doing something special, or leaving our familiar settings behind. But relaxation isn't just time at the beach. In fact, some people come back from vacation more fatigued than before they left. But you can relax without stepping outside your own house. In fact, relaxation can be most profound when you seek it right where you are now.

The Relaxation Response

One kind of relaxation that's popular today is the *relaxation response*, a simple method popularized by Herbert Benson, M.D., at the Harvard Medical School.[3] Although ancient in origin, the relaxation response has been the subject of dozens of scientific studies over several decades that have confirmed its benefits. So what is it, exactly? The relaxation response is a state of mental calm during which your blood pressure drops, your heart and breathing rates slow, and your muscles become less tense. Attaining this state of physical and mental calm is simple, and it has many benefits that range from coping better with stress, feeling more at ease with yourself, and living more fully "in the moment."

Here's how Dr. Benson describes the method of using this technique:

- Sit quietly in a comfortable position.

- Close your eyes.

- Deeply relax all your muscles, beginning at your feet and progressing upward to your face. Keep them relaxed.

- Breathe through your nose. Become aware of your breathing. As you breathe out, say the word "one" silently to yourself. For example, breathe in . . . out, *one,* in . . . out, *one,* and so forth. Breathe easily and naturally.

- Continue this pattern for 10 to 20 minutes. You may open your eyes to check the time, but don't use an alarm. When you finish, sit quietly for several minutes, at first with your eyes closed and later with your eyes open. Don't stand up for a few minutes.

- Don't worry about whether you are "successful" in achieving a deep level of relaxation. Maintain a passive attitude, and permit relaxation to occur at its own pace. When distracting thoughts occur, try to ignore them by not dwelling upon them and return to repeating *one.*

With practice, the relaxation response should come with little effort. Practice the technique once or twice daily, but not within two hours after any meal, since the digestive processes seem to interfere with the elicitation of the relaxation response.

Progressive Relaxation

At Structure House, we teach a variety of methods for relaxation and stress relief that our participants find helpful in coping with weight loss issues, health problems, and aspects of daily life. One such method is *progressive relaxation*, a technique for reducing tension through body awareness.[4]

Here's an example of progressive relaxation. Trying it even once may surprise you—you'll realize how much tension you routinely carry around. Just follow this simple sequence of steps:

- Position yourself on a chair in whatever way you find comfortable; however, it's important for your back to be straight. (Some people prefer to do relaxation exercises lying down, and that's fine, but keep in mind that it's easy to doze off when you're in a reclining position.)

- Sit comfortably with your back straight. The height of the chair should be such that your knees are approximately level with the height of your hips.

- Sit straight and toward the back of the chair. Make sure that your lower back is pushed in so that your back is straight. You feet should be roughly a shoulder's width apart. Your hands can rest palms-down on your thighs.

- Note any discomfort. If you feel uncomfortable, you may need to adjust your position slightly, but you'll find that the position will become more comfortable over time.

- Squeeze your hands gently into fists. Take a few moments to really feel the tension. Then, after a few seconds, release all the tension in your hands.

- Pause for a moment. Notice the difference between the state of tension you felt earlier and the state of relaxation you feel now. Feeling this difference is the basis of this progressive relaxation technique.

- Now go through the same sequence with your feet and hands at the same time. Gently curl your toes and clench your hands into fists. Hold that tension for a few seconds, then let go, releasing the tension completely.

- Repeat the process again, this time tensing your upper and lower legs along with your toes and hands. Feel the tension for a moment. Then release the tightness in all those muscles, letting them relax completely.

- Now repeat the process again, this time tensing your shoulders toward your ears and scrunching all your face muscles together as if wincing in pain; simultaneously, tense your upper and lower legs along with your toes and hands. Feel the tension again for a moment. Then release the tightness in all those muscles, letting them relax completely.

- Within a few minutes, all the tension in your body will have dissipated, leaving you feeling more relaxed and peaceful.

Mindfulness

Another technique taught widely at Structure House is *mindfulness*. This is a type of meditation that is derived from ancient wisdom traditions and predates more recent variations like the relaxation response. Mindfulness is the art of becoming deeply aware of the present moment— fully experiencing what happens in the here and now. The purpose of mindfulness is to awaken consciousness. It's a technique for focusing your mind on what's happening in and around you at a given moment. Mindfulness is important because it helps you live more fully rather than letting your experiences rush past, something that has become all too easy in our high-pressure modern life. This technique helps you turn down all the noise in your head—the anger, frustration, anxiety, doubt, and self-blame that may be distracting, fatiguing, and upsetting you from moment to moment.[5]

Here's how mindfulness works. The key isn't so much *what you focus on* but *how you focus*. At the heart of mindfulness is the quality of the awareness you bring to each moment. By paying closer attention in this manner, you become more *present to* and *aware of* both the inner and outer experiences of life as it unfolds. Mindfulness is a silent witness, accepting and nonjudgmental, of your experience. I want to emphasize, however, that calling mindfulness "accepting and nonjudgmental" does *not* mean that mindfulness advocates withdrawal from commitment to the world. Rather, mindfulness teaches you to acknowledge your moment-to-moment reality and prepares you to respond to that reality less impulsively and more effectively. As your awareness of the unfolding present moment intensifies and clarifies, so does your capacity to live more fully and to deal with the world more effectively. It's a form of training that allows you to *be with* what is already here by letting go of any unnecessary tendencies to "hold on."

Here are the seven essential attributes of mindfulness:

- **Nonjudgment.** Mindfulness encourages being an impartial witness to your own experience. Try to increase your awareness of thinking as it arises, with attention focused on the quality of your mind states. Simply note that thinking or judging is present. Don't judge the judging!

- **Patience.** We all have a tendency to rush from one moment of experience to the next, often with little attention paid to what we are experiencing. Mindfulness encourages patience—a form of wisdom that allows us to recognize that experience must unfold in its own time.

- **Openness.** By habit and cultural training, we tend to prejudge, categorize, and analyze experiences rather than truly living them in the here and now. Mindfulness encourages "beginner's mind"—an openness to direct experience of what's happening, an acceptance of what the senses provide, and receptivity to whatever arises as a unique and precious event. This approach leaves you less burdened by expectations based on past experiences and more open to new possibilities.

- **Trust.** Mindfulness means taking responsibility for being yourself—learning to listen to and trust your own being. Can you listen to your feelings and intuitions? Can you let yourself grow and change? Through mindfulness, you can practice turning toward experience with an increased sense of safety and trust.

- **Nonstriving.** Because mindfulness emphasizes close attention to whatever is happening, it stresses *being* rather than *doing*. There's a paradox within meditative practice: the best way to achieve your goals of stress reduction, personal development, or spiritual growth is to back off from striving for results. Instead, focus carefully on seeing and accepting things as they are (and how they change) from moment to moment. *Striving less* and *being more* can evoke new ways of experiencing ourselves and the world around us.

- **Acceptance.** Mindfulness encourages you to see things *as they are* rather than *as you think they ought to be.* We're all subject to complex, often intense preconceptions about the nature of reality. We waste a lot of time and energy denying or resisting what is already in play, trying to force events to fit our own expectations. By contrast, mindfulness nudges us toward accepting things as they are *in this moment* as a precondition for change.

- **Nonattachment.** We habitually cling to ideas and views about ourselves and others. Mindfulness advocates nonattachment—a willingness to let go of the urge to elevate some aspects of our experience and reject other aspects. This process of letting go helps us to accept our experience as it is, moment by moment.

An Exercise in Mindfulness

The mindfulness tradition encompasses a multiplicity of practices, among them sitting meditation, walking meditation, and many others. What follows is just one of the many popular forms of practice within this tradition.

- Sit comfortably on a pad, cushion, or chair. If you're sitting on a pad or cushion, cross your legs loosely in front of you. Your knees should be lower than your hips. If you're sitting on a chair, sit straight without leaning against the chair's back.

- Rest your hands comfortably on your thighs, or else cup your palms (the right hand in the left) and rest them on your lap.

- Keep your back straight, but without straining.

- Position your head by means of a level gaze ahead.

- Let your eyes close without squeezing them shut.

- Relax your jaw and mouth, leaving your teeth slightly apart.

- Rest the tip of your tongue behind your upper front teeth.

- Breathe in and out gently, never forcing the breath.

- As you exhale, note the sensation of the air passing through your nostrils, or else note the air leaving the tip of your nostrils.

- Focus gently on your breath as you inhale and exhale. Observe your breath.

- As you breathe, many thoughts and feelings will arise, distracting you from your breath. Simply observe these thoughts and feelings without judgment; allow them to pass. Don't get caught up in the "story" of the thought. Simply and gently return your awareness once again, over and over, to your breath.

- Physical sensations—joint pains, itches, twitches—may arise as you sit. Note these sensations and, to the degree possible, consider them without judgment and without responding to them. Simply be aware of your body.

- Continue this process for about 20 minutes at first, then longer (up to 45 minutes) as you grow more familiar and comfortable with the practice.

- As you continue to sit and breathe, try to steep in the present moment as if in calm water, absorbing it into your being.

Note that there is no "destination" for this practice—no transcendent state of mind you're striving for, no mystical experience. The journey itself is the destination; the process itself is the goal.

Mindfulness and Structured Eating

You can see the implications for Structured Eating. We often rush our meals and eat as if on autopilot. It's common for people to eat while watching TV, reading the paper, or working at the computer—and sometimes doing all three at once! I speak to many people at Structure House who say that they "graze" or just "fill up," as if they're cows or cars. Many people eat—and often overeat—without paying much attention to the food in front of them. In this way, you miss out on the experience of eating.

In comparison to these half-oblivious states of filling up or chowing down, mindful eating encourages you to focus on the full experience of your food—the richness of the flavors, the subtlety of the aromas, the variety of the textures, and all the other aspects of eating that are pleasurable to the senses. Sometimes Structure House participants express worry that becoming so aware of their food will tempt them to overeat even more. I believe that the opposite is more likely. If you take your time while eating; if your process of consuming your meal is something you experience moment by moment; if you're truly aware of what you're doing at the table—then I believe that mindfulness will leave you more satisfied and *less* likely to overeat.

Mindful eating avoids the rush of compulsive eating and encourages a slower, more fully focused, more enriching experience—a meal consumed as a series of fully savored moments. Being more fully present with your self and your body while eating is a powerful way to explore a healthier relationship with food. For instance, Dr. Jon Kabat-Zinn, a proponent of mindfulness, hands each of his students a single raisin and asks them to eat it as an exercise in mindfulness. I think you'd agree that most of us would simply pop the raisin in our mouth, chew a few times, and swallow, all without paying much attention, except perhaps to want more. But mindful eating—even when eating a single raisin—is much different.

Here's a similar exercise you can try, this one using a tangerine as the object of mindfulness.

- Take the tangerine and hold it in your hand. Is it cool, neutral in temperature, or warm to the touch? Is it soft or firm? What does the surface feel like—leather, plastic, something else?

- Look at it closely. Is it uniformly orange? Uneven? Flawed or unflawed?

- Examine the tangerine as if you've never encountered one before. Wonder about it—what it is, where it came from.

- Now smell the tangerine. Does it have a scent, or is it odorless?

- Notice any urges to eat it—any sense of impatience, thoughts, feelings, or desires.

- Holding the fruit in one hand, push into the skin with the other hand's thumb or fingers and pull open the tangerine. What does that effort feel like . . . and does the skin resist your touch or open easily? Does it make a sound as you peel it back? What does the fruit smell like now? Savor the scent.

- Peel the tangerine. Feel the damp lining of the skin. Look at the spiral you've pulled away from the fruit inside. Squeeze the peel and smell the little spritz of citrus oil it produces.

- Be aware of your conscious decision to eat this food. Note any thoughts or feelings. . . . Do you feel any sense of excitement?

- Now pull apart the little segments of tangerine and put one in your mouth. What does it taste like before you bite down? Now bite into the segment. How does the flavor change? Is it sweet, tart, or both?

- Chew it slowly. Notice the textures—how they change as the juice comes out and the segment empties.

- Does this tangerine evoke any feelings or memories? (One person recalled a trip to Spain and the tangerine trees growing in her hotel's garden. Another recalled experiences of Christmas during his boyhood, when tangerines were a rare seasonal treat.) Practice being aware of the distinctions between the sensations in the moment and all the thoughts and feelings evoked by the act of eating.

- Chew and swallow, feeling the pulp go down your throat and esophagus all the way to your stomach.

- Gradually eat the rest of the tangerine, noticing sensations and thoughts as you proceed. See if you can taste each bite as fully as the first. Notice any changes in taste, any changes in sensations of hunger or satisfaction of your appetite.

- Once you've finished eating the tangerine, pause and reflect on the experience. Notice any thoughts of "wanting more" or any feelings of "having enough." What else can you be aware of before your transition to your next activity?

Mindful eating, like mindfulness in general, is not a panacea. As a way of being fully present to your own experience, however, it can make each meal a richer (and more enriching) experience. A deeper awareness of each moment—including the moments when you happen to be eating—

will help to satisfy appetites that go beyond the physiological appetite for food.

Once you've gathered and mastered the use of your tools, you can build a stronger house and you will be able to make all the necessary repairs for the years to come.

CHAPTER 10

Explore Lifestyle Change

"Taking good care of yourself will change the path of your life—and in a positive, rewarding way. Fulfilling and wonderful. And it enhances every aspect of your life. It's important to view self-care in a broader sense than just eating. Self-care is just as vital. In addition to eating, it's fitness, it's being true to yourself. If you need to say no to a friend, say no to a friend. Those kinds of things."

—Lisa

"[Self-care is] getting in touch with who you are. Not who others think you ought to be, but who you are. What makes you happy. What brings joy to your life. Let people know that you love them and support them, but it's not your job to fix them. You're working on fixing yourself."

—Sallie

"My experience was, I needed to change my lifestyle. I was traveling two hundred days a year. That didn't work for me in letting go of the weight. And I really needed to get rooted and grounded."

—Peter

Earlier in this book, I stated that I want you to do more than just change your diet; I want you to change your life. Weight loss and improved health are certainly admirable goals in their own right. However, you'll attain more substantial success in reaching these goals if you consider some issues that go beyond how many calories you consume each day and what number you see on the scale when you weigh yourself.

I'm referring in part to your relationship with food—an issue we've discussed throughout the book. What are the antecedents, or "eating triggers," that prompt your Unstructured Eating? To what degree can you change your responses to these antecedents? One part of the Structure House program is certainly to look at and change your relationship with food. But that relationship with food *happens in a context:* habit, boredom, and stress don't occur without any connection with what takes place in the rest of your life. For this reason, a crucial part of the Structure House program is to look at your lifestyle in a more general sense.

I am amused by programs that speak of dealing with "lifestyle." When I look at their definitions of "lifestyle," I see that it is usually the idea of eating less and exercising more. But lifestyle extends far beyond those two issues. That was why, when I founded Structure House in 1977, I called our facility Structure House Center for Weight Control and Lifestyle Change.

LIFESTYLE CHANGE—THE WRAPPER
AND THE CONTENTS

What I'm suggesting is that you look more closely at certain aspects of your life, think about what you do and why you do it, and challenge some of the ways in which our culture may influence your perception of yourself.

In part, I am also referring to the way you use your time. Recall that the Structure House Diary opens to two pages: on the left, food use, and on the right, time. How you spend your time is critical. What I'm presenting here is a way in which you can look at how you spend your time. Remember: your time is going to be spent somehow. That's a guarantee. Either you can *decide how you're going to make things happen*—or you can *simply let things happen to you.*

One way to consider these issues is to view them from the standpoint of the *wrapper* and the *contents*. In this image, the wrapper is the surface reasons that prompt your concern about overweight and health issues. You see the number on the scale, so you decide to lose weight. You see your blood pressure readout on the dial, so you decide to reduce your blood pressure. You feel winded after five minutes on the treadmill, so you decide to improve your level of fitness. These are all important issues to address. By trying to lose weight, lower your blood pressure, and improve your fitness, you're acknowledging that something is out of balance and you're trying to regain it. But *what* is out of balance? Is it simply your diet? Your sodium intake? Your level of exercise? Or is the imbalance something more profound? Perhaps something deeper than just the *wrapper*—the surface reasons—is causing the imbalance you perceive. What are the deeper satisfactions and dissatisfactions in your life? What is the real quality of your experience—the true depth of meaning that goes beyond the surface aspects?

These questions lead us to consider the *contents:* the deeper issues you face. I urge you to consider asking some questions that address these deeper issues:

- Are you willing to engage in an ongoing exploration of your fundamental attitudes and beliefs?
- Where are you in your life cycle, and what are your needs at this point in your life?
- What does it mean to explore not just external but also internal aspects of life—the quality of life, a sense of meaning and satisfaction?
- At the end of your life, whenever that may occur, what is it going to mean to you?

Asking these questions is challenging. It means going beyond the surface issues of what you eat and what you weigh to much more subtle issues of what you want your life to be. It's challenging to explore what lies beneath the surface. It's challenging to accept that you're accomplished in your work but that your accomplishments pressure you to use food as a "relief valve" to compensate for stress and fatigue. It's challenging to admit that you pay a high price by neglecting self-care, relationships, and personal life. It's challenging to explore your deepest attitudes and to start making changes in what you do and how you perceive yourself.

To help you in this process, this chapter offers some "lenses" that can help you see your life more clearly—and see some new possibilities for making changes and accepting the benefits of change. If you can accept these possibilities, you can gain a perspective on life that's less automatic and more considered, one that offers you more options as you choose what you want to do and be. In short, you can engage with life in a healthier way.

To foster this process, let's focus on three primary issues: *balance, active leisure,* and *healthy pleasures.* Each of these is important in its own right. In addition, they connect directly to some of the issues we've discussed in other chapters, such as stress management, other coping skills, and finding replacements for unstructured eating. Each of these topics also addresses these questions:

First, how can you start to build a lifestyle that acknowledges the full range of your needs as a human being—including the needs for rewards, for relaxation, for pleasure, and for nurturance?

And second, how can you meet these needs in ways that are less dependent on food?

TASK 1: LOOK FOR BALANCE IN YOUR LIFE

Many Structure House participants are heard to say, "Something is out of balance" or "My life is unbalanced." Sometimes they can identify the problem that's affecting them: "I feel so weighed down by responsibilities that I try to shift the balance by eating." At other times they don't know what's out of balance, but they know there's a problem. They understand that part of what drives them to Unstructured Eating is an imbalance between obligations and leisure, between work and play, between stress and relaxation, between exertion and rest. In response to these several kinds of imbalance, they use food as a tranquilizer, as a way of quenching anger, and as a consolation for unmet emotional needs. Food is a multipurpose "tool" for addressing these various issues of stress, boredom, and loneliness. You can use food to replace whatever's missing or to address whatever is off balance.

But does Unstructured Eating really address these issues of balance?

In response to the situation I'm describing, part of examining your lifestyle is to consider *what sorts of balance exist in your day-to-day life* and, in addition, *what might be out of balance.* Understanding issues of balance and imbalance provides opportunities to address commitments and activities that may be weighing on you and prompting Unstructured Eating. Examining these issues may also help you identify healthier ways to reward and nurture yourself—to express your wants and needs in noncaloric ways.

"Balance Is a Luxury I Can't Afford"

When I raise the issue of balance, many people respond by acknowledging the problem but also by stating that there's nothing to be done about it. A typical response is "I know my life is out of control, but that's just how it goes" or "Balance is a luxury I can't really afford—I'm doing the best I can just to muddle through." I also hear genuine, heartfelt explanations of why gaining a better sense of balance isn't possible: "I have to focus completely on my career" or "I'm a single mom" or "My family needs so much attention from me" or "My parents are old and sick." I sympathize with all these dilemmas. I'm certainly aware that everyone faces complex family and work issues and that many people struggle with genuine hardships. However, I'm concerned that people see so few options before them. Is balance truly a luxury they can't afford? Wouldn't it be better to take a step back, examine what may have gone wrong, and be open to previously unnoticed choices and opportunities?

Here's why being open-minded about balance is so important: You can't simply expend energy all the time; you have to refuel as well. You understandably feel fatigued and stressed by life's demands. But is it advisable—or even possible—to run on empty? Not for long. If you ignore your own needs for physical and emotional replenishment, even your best-intentioned efforts will grind to a halt. Ironically, attending to your own needs may be one of the best things you can do for others. Taking twenty minutes to exercise, meditate, or just sit and listen to music may be exactly what you need to regain your energy, well-being, and patience—which in turn may be exactly what you need to give more attention to the people who are dependent on you. How can you be present for other people if you don't take care of yourself?

In response to this situation, I want you to be your own lifestyle coach—your own consultant. I want you to look at how you spend your time and how you balance your activities. I want you to ask yourself, "What gets in the way of my being more skillful with myself in my own life?" If you can observe yourself with a little objectivity, I bet you'll have a good sense of what to do. You probably have great insights and wisdom about how to be more skillful. Being as objective as possible, look at your life. Observe what's working well and what's not. What do you want to retain in your life? And what do you want to let go of?

Here's an approach you may find helpful.

"Ought-tos" and "Want-tos"

Consider how you spend your time. Look at each hour of the day—or, better yet, sample a sequence of days to look for patterns—to get an overview of your activities and where they fit into your life. The worksheet on page 224 can help you assess these activities, ask questions about them, and reach insights about how they influence your thoughts, your emotions, and your actions.

- How are you spending your time and energy?
- Which activities cause you to feel dissatisfaction, stress, and fatigue?
- Which grant you a sense of fulfillment, relief, and completion?
- Which create an impulse toward nonnutritive eating?
- What times of day leave you vulnerable to food use?

Look at the Balance Assessment chart on page 224. To gain a clearer sense of how you use your time—and how your activities may prompt Unstructured Eating—just follow these steps:

Balance Assessment

Time	Activity	Work	Relationships	Self-care	"Want-to" versus "Ought-to"					Pleasure	Relaxation/ Renewal	Meaning/ Satisfaction	Food Use	Notes
hour	(describe)		(choose a category)		(rate from 1	2	3	4	or 5)		(choose a category)		(antecedents)	
	TOTALS													TOTALS

1. Under "Time," log the day's activities, starting when you wake.

2. Under "Activity," briefly indicate the important aspects of what you're doing, who you're with, or where you are. You can use more than one line, if necessary. Examples: "Bkfst w/kids—kitchen"; "commute—stuck in traffic"; "work—mtngs; 2 hrs."

3. For "Work"/"Relationships"/"Self-care," put a checkmark or an X for the category of your activity.

4. For "Want-to"/"Ought-to," rate (on a scale of 1 to 5) whether you feel that you *want* to be doing this activity or you *ought* to be doing it. Do you feel a sense of investment, satisfaction, delight, commitment, and completion from this activity? Or, instead, do you feel dread, frustration, or stress? One is the greatest degree of "Want-to"; 5 is the greatest degree of "Ought-to." Note: don't rate sleep, which will skew your ratings and give a distorted picture of your overall balance.

5. Under the columns labeled "Pleasure," "Relaxation/Renewal," and "Meaning/Satisfaction," put a checkmark or an X if one or more apply. Here again, don't rate the hours you spend asleep.

6. Note any food use (Unstructured Eating) associated with specific activities you've listed. Perhaps you munch snack foods to deal with the stress of your commute, or perhaps you habitually eat a bowl of ice cream to unwind after work.

7. Once you've filled out a page for a given period—usually a single day—total up your activities and evaluations. (Better yet, examine a week, a month, or an even longer period of time.) How many checkmarks (or Xs) have you accumulated for Work, how many for Relationships, and how many for Self-care? What is the pattern of 1's, 2's, 3's, 4's, and 5's under the "Want-to"/"Ought-to" scale? How many activities inspired a sense of Pleasure, Relaxation/Renewal, or Meaning/Satisfaction? How many activities—and which ones—have prompted Unstructured Eating? Finally, what times of day (or times of the week or of a particular time of year, such as during holidays or vacations) are high-risk times for Unstructured Eating?

I need to comment further about the issue of "Ought-tos" and "Want-tos."

The "Ought-to" category includes all those activities or actions that you regard as *obligations* or *sources of stress*—experiences or tasks that prompt a feeling of burden or dread as you anticipate them on your calendar. These are the things you just *have to* or *ought to* get done. Ought-tos tend to leave you feeling depleted or stressed. They use up your energy rather than energizing you. If your life is heavily imbalanced with Ought-tos, you may feel that your world has narrowed or become more negative; you may feel more obsessive, critical, isolated, or disconnected; or you may feel a diminished sense of self-esteem.

By contrast, "Want-tos" are aspects of life that are *replenishing*. They provide replenishment, renewal, and a sense of relief. They are activities and tasks that you look forward to and derive satisfaction from; they inspire a sense of excitement when you see them on the calendar; they leave you feeling uplifted and reenergized. An abundance of Want-tos may even change your perspective or worldview, so that you feel more optimistic, capable, empowered, and in control, with a higher sense of self-esteem and a greater sense of belonging or connection with your family, your coworkers, your community, or the world.

Many Ought-tos and Want-tos inspire similar reactions from most people; others prompt more individual responses. Most people would feel that cleaning up a messy backyard is an Ought-to, while playing a favorite sport is a Want-to. However, personal preferences enter into many other perceptions of what is energy-draining and what is energy-renewing. *What constitutes an "Ought-to" activity versus a "Want-to" activity is highly individual.* Some people would rather putter in a yard than play a sport. Some people enjoy cooking; others find it unpleasant or stressful. Some people like fixing car problems; others find it unpleasant or stressful. Some people enjoy playing with toddlers; others find it unpleasant or stressful. In filling out the worksheet, the core issue isn't an abstract notion of Ought-to and Want-to; it's what *you* feel you ought to do versus what you want to do.

So use the chart to track a given day—or duplicate it to chart a series of days. (You can rely on your memory; you can transfer data from your Structure House Diary; or you can do both.) How are you spending your twenty-four hours—"spending" in terms of both the *amount of time spent* and *the quality of the time spent*? What are your activities? Which of them are Ought-tos and which are Want-tos? What are these activities when categorized according to Work, Relationships, and Self-care? How "extreme" are these activities on the numbered scale (1, 2, 3, 4, 5—with 1 representing the most extreme Ought-to and 5 representing the most extreme Want-to)? Which activities have given you a sense of pleasure, relaxation/renewal, or meaning/satisfaction? Note those as well. At the end of the day, how many activities count as Ought-tos and how many as Want-tos? Also, note which activities have happened before or during episodes of Unstructured Eating.

As you look at these examples and how they stack up as Ought-tos and Want-tos, try to evaluate the situation as if you were viewing someone else's life. Sit back and pretend you're this person's lifestyle coach. Let's say that your activities are heavy on Ought-tos and light on Want-tos. What is the pattern you see between Ought-to activities and Unstructured Eating? Given the imbalance between Ought-tos and Want-tos, what is your food use going to look like at the end of the day if you're expending more energy than you're replenishing? I think it's safe to say that you won't feel so great. You'll feel depleted, drained, and running on empty. This exercise can also be useful as a way of revealing the connections among these three factors:

- Where and how you're spending your time
- The impact of those activities on your life
- The consequences in terms of Unstructured Eating

Now look at the Balance Assessment Examples chart on page 228. This is the same chart, but now it's filled out with responses typical of how many of us live our lives nowadays. Tracking a twenty-four-hour period from 6 A.M. one morning to 5 A.M. the next, the activities listed are heavy on time devoted to work (11 hours' worth), light on relationships (4), and almost nonexistent on self-care (2). There's also a heavy preponderance of Ought-tos over Want-tos. pleasure, relaxation/renewal, and meaning/satisfaction are present—but not in abundance. Is it surprising that the lack of balance revealed here has led to lots of antecedents (heavy on stress) and in turn to plenty of Unstructured Eating? Not at all.

Consider this scenario. Marissa spends at least an hour and a half each morning on her commute to work, then at least that long coming home each evening. The loss of time is annoying in its own right. In addition, she has to deal with the stress of traffic, repeated close calls with aggressive drivers, and the boredom of being stuck in her car. This situation unquestionably falls into the Ought-to category; it causes Marissa a lot of stress;

Balance Assessment Examples

Time	Activity	Work	Relationships	Self-care	"Want-to" (rate from 1)	2	3	4	"Ought-to" (or 5)	Pleasure	Relaxation/Renewal	Meaning/Satisfaction	Food Use	Notes
hour	(describe)		(choose a category)								(choose a category)		(antecedents)	
6:00 A.M.	shower/BR			X		X					X			
7:00 A.M.	bkfst w/ kids		X									X	habit	extra food!
8:00 A.M.	commute/traffic	X						X					stress	munchies
9:00 A.M.	work crisis mode	X							X				stress	
10:00 A.M.	2-hr. meeting	X							X					
11:00 A.M.	2-hr. meeting	X							X					
Noon	bus. lunch	X							X				stress/snacks	doughnuts
1:00 P.M.	project work	X							X			X	habit/stress	big portions
2:00 P.M.	project work	X					X							
3:00 P.M.	project work	X						X						
4:00 P.M.	meeting	X						X	X				stress/fatigue	candy bar
5:00 P.M.	meeting	X							X					
6:00 P.M.	commute/traffic	X							X				boredom	cola
7:00 P.M.	dinner at home		X			X							habit	munchies
8:00 P.M.	kid care/bedtime		X			X				X		X	stress/fatigue	ate extra
9:00 P.M.	kid care/bedtime		X			X				X		X		
10:00 P.M.	TV/hanging out			X		X						X	habit	chips
11:00 P.M.	sleep													
Midnight	sleep													
1:00 A.M.	sleep													
2:00 A.M.	sleep													
3:00 A.M.	sleep													
4:00 A.M.	sleep													
5:00 A.M.	sleep													
	TOTALS	11	4	2		5	4	4	8	2	2	4	9	TOTALS

and it often leads to Unstructured Eating—out of boredom while in the car (such as munching on cookies or doughnuts) and as stress relief afterward (such as binging when she gets home). Totaling up her activities, Marissa sees that she is carrying a heavy load of Ought-tos, and her commute is one of the most frustrating and depleting of all.

But let's move beyond the obvious frustration that Marissa faces and consider how she might deal with it. What are her possibilities for coping with the time-wasting, stressful aspects of her commute?

First of all, let's ask whether this daily three-hour commute is really necessary. Marissa's answer may be "Yes. I like my job too much to quit, and I like where I live too much to move. These two places are almost fifty miles apart, so I'm stuck with the commute." Because of her commitment to staying in a town with good schools and a high quality of life, Marissa is willing to put up with the hassles of commuting. But commutes are notoriously a time of high stress and dissatisfaction—a situation that can lead to a high degree of Unstructured Eating. So if Marissa is committed to keeping her commute, how can she cope with it so that she's not tempted to eat so much either during or after each leg of the commute?

One strategy would be to use that time differently. Some possibilities: Marissa could listen to music CDs, books on tape, or even language instruction CDs in the car. The goal is to make that time more palatable and less stressful. These are all ways to reduce the *intensity* of what she's experiencing.

Another strategy would be to reduce the *frequency* of this Ought-to situation. Perhaps Marissa could reduce her commute from five days a week to three or four by switching to a part-time schedule or by working at home a day or two per week. Alternatively, she might use public transportation instead of driving, which would enable her to read en route to work instead of fighting the traffic.

Still another approach would be to examine the wider context—what we might call the *frame* around the issue of Marissa's commute. She had decided that putting up with her commute is important and tolerable this year, since her son, Jared, is a senior at the local high school. Staying in their town is currently a top priority. But once this year is over and Jared heads off to college, Marissa and her husband can reevaluate their decision to stay put. It's possible that moving closer to her job—or moving to a different community—will be options at that time, which would help to ease her commute-related stress.

Any of these approaches might help her lessen the impact of this stress. Or she might be able to balance the Ought-to activity with one that's more of a Want-to. In short, she can create a better balance.

The Nature of Balance

To understand balance, it's important to recognize its effects on three main areas of life: (1) work, (2) relationships and support, and (3) self-care. Being out of balance in any of these areas can be an antecedent of Unstructured Eating.

- **Work.** "Work" doesn't necessarily mean what you do for money; rather, it's what you do to provide yourself with a sense of skill, mastery, purpose, meaning, and productivity. It might be a job or a career, but it could also be an avocation, hobby, or volunteer activity.

- **Relationships and support.** We human beings are social, interactive creatures. We need certain things from other people: love, attention, approval, touch, information, advice, encouragement, and mentoring. Adequate interpersonal support can help us feel less stress, which can translate into better health and longevity. Support can also help people maintain success in weight control.

- **Self-care.** We also need to nurture ourselves. We help ourselves from within by knowing how to relax and by giving ourselves encouragement and self-acknowledgment. Good attitudes and positive self-talk are important as ways of diverting yourself, distracting yourself, and providing yourself with comfort. Self-care includes good nutrition, physical activity, grooming, getting enough sleep, and providing yourself with activities that connect you to a sense of meaning—whether by means of contemplation, prayer, community, or spirituality.

Note that the realms of work, relationships, and self-care don't exist in isolation; on the contrary, they are closely interrelated. Overdoing one aspect of life, such as work, usually means that you'll end up underdoing another aspect of life, such as self-care or relationships. It's possible to overdo or underdo in any of these three areas—work, relationships, and self-care. But "overdoing" and "underdoing" aren't just a matter of the time spent; overdoing and underdoing are also affected by the *substance* of what you're doing and the *emotional content* of what's happening.

Suppose you spend several hours each night focusing on family activities. You hang out with your children, you help them with their homework, you get them ready for bed. These activities require an output of your energy, but they energize you, too, because you enjoy your family's time together. But when you look more closely at those evening hours, what's actually happening? You're answering the phone, you're getting ready for some work-related tasks tomorrow, and you're paying bills while simultaneously answering your children's questions about long division or the Revolutionary War. Multitasking tends to distract you and disrupt your potential for experiencing satisfaction and meaning during that family time. The stress that situations like these produce can become the antecedent of Unstructured food use—in this case, evening snacks that serve as a "safety valve" during a time when you are in demand to meet others' needs.

Situations like these are a reality that we all face. The bottom line is that even if you strive for balance, it's difficult to attain it. So how can you assess imbalances in your life and then try to address them?

Evaluate Your "Pie of Life"

One of the easiest ways to size up balance is what many people call the "Pie of Life." This simple pie chart allows you to see the proportions (or disproportions) of work, relationships, and self-care in your life in black and white.

Here's how to create and use the Pie of Life.

First, take a blank sheet of paper. Draw a large circle on the page. Now, using information you acquired earlier by listing your Ought-tos and Want-tos on the worksheet, divide the pie into segments that are proportional to the total time devoted to work, relationships and support, and self-care. (As before, don't count the time you're asleep. Although sleep is certainly a crucial aspect of self-care, listing the hours you spend asleep will skew your numbers and provide a distorted picture of your situation. That said, you should generally take sleep into account in other evaluations of balance.) If you work a standard eight-hour workday, your job accounts for a third of the twenty-four-hour day, so the wedge alloted to work should be a third of the whole pie. If you work a twelve-hour workday, the "work" wedge should be half of the pie.

Life in Balance

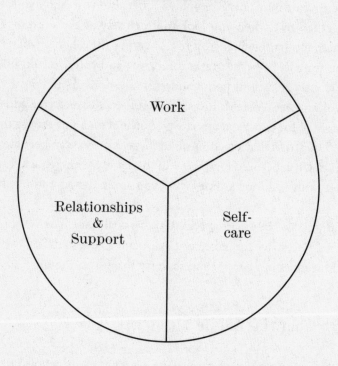

Mike, a 39-year-old paralegal, used the Pie of Life to get an overview of balance. The results showed that Mike devotes 80 percent of his time to work, 10 percent to relationships, and 10 percent to self-care. He has known for years that he feels "out of whack," as he puts it, and he has assumed that spending too much time at the office is part of the problem. Mike has also been aware that his long hours at work lead to stress and fatigue that he "treats" by Unstructured Eating. Similarly, the lack of enough satisfying time with other people prompts him to fill the void of his loneliness with food. But he didn't visualize the situation clearly until he did the Pie of Life exercise. Now the evidence of imbalance is right in front of him.

Mike Out of Balance

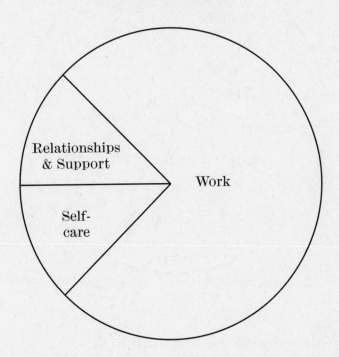

The big question now is what to do about it. The answer isn't a quick fix. My suggestion: Mike should gradually reduce his time at the office by 10 to 20 percent—ideally to a total of about 60 percent—and he should add 5 to 10 percent of his time to each of the relationships and self-care categories. Will this "adjustment" resolve the imbalance in his life? That's impossible to answer definitively. These three steps can be challenging, and their benefits are incremental, but they will head Mike in the right direction—not only by addressing the issue of balance but also by easing his temptation to use Unstructured Eating as a primary way of coping. Ideally, Mike will also begin to explore *why* his life is out of balance. (His personal circumstances happen to include a divorce several years ago.)

Addressing the balance in his life will also raise some deeper issues of satisfaction and meaning:

Mike Strives for Balance

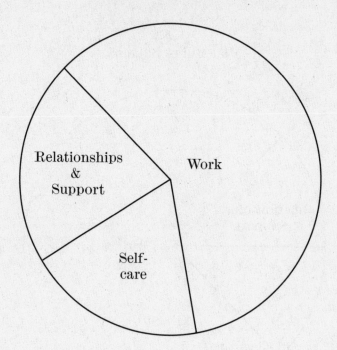

- How did Mike's overwork-oriented lifestyle take shape?
- To what degree does his tendency to spend long hours at the office indicate an effort to avoid intimacy?
- To what degree is his Unstructured Eating a response to loneliness?
- What would he have to do to "live into" a more balanced life?
- Is he willing to say "yes" to the benefits of a more balanced life?
- Is he willing to understand how his *resistance* to a more balanced life has included its own payoffs? (For instance, his overwork has led to some success in business—though at considerable personal cost.)
- Is he willing to take the risks associated with investing time and effort in relationships—even if that means deemphasizing his career goals to some extent?
- Can he accept himself as a worthy person if he redefines himself *less in terms of his work role* and *more in terms of nonwork activities and commitments*?
- Can he tolerate the challenge of allowing other people into his life and accepting the uncertainty inherent in new relationships?

I would certainly never claim that such questions can be answered quickly. Dealing with issues of these sorts and taking steps toward a more balanced life are major challenges. But asking the questions and considering the answers are necessary first steps in working toward change.

Examine Myths that Affect Balance

Some unexamined beliefs or attitudes in our culture may become obstacles to living a more balanced life. I call these beliefs and attitudes "myths" because they're so ingrained and pervasive, and because they're often at odds with the nature of reality. Some of these myths may sound extreme—statements that you perceive as unrealistic or impractical—yet they may influence you on an emotional level. They may contribute to the situation that faces most people: puzzlement over the gap between, on the one hand, *what you know makes sense*; and, on the other hand, *what you actually do*. Or, as many Structure House participants put it, "How is it possible that I know what I ought to do, but I consistently find myself not doing it?" Ask yourself to what degree you're subscribing to the following myths:

Myths About Selfishness and Selflessness

- To take care of my family, I must be very successful in my work.
- To be successful in work, I must make tremendous personal sacrifices.
- To be a good parent, I must always put everyone else ahead of myself.
- To be a competent professional, I must deny my personal needs.
- If I attend to my emotional life, it shows that I'm weak and self-indulgent.
- At the point when life's demands ease, *then* I can take care of my needs.

The Reality of Selfishness and Selflessness

Taking care of your family and being successful at work may not have any direct cause-effect relationship. In fact, personal sacrifices (at work or elsewhere) may complicate rather than improve your efforts to achieve success. Ignoring your personal needs may actually damage your professional competence. Far from being weak and self-indulgent, attending to your emotional needs may strengthen you and make you more responsive to others. Life's demands never really ease; if you wait for that day, you'll probably wait forever.

Myths About Relaxation
- Relaxation is nothing more than the absence of stress or the reduction of stress.
- To relax, all you have to do is kick back and let it happen.
- Relaxing and collapsing are essentially the same thing.

The Reality of Relaxation
Relaxation isn't simply the absence of stress, and the absence of stress is incompatible with life. In reality, you need to plan for, create, and defend the time and place to relax. Collapsing doesn't feel good or restore your sense of self.

Myths About Play
- Play is just for children.
- Play is nothing more than having fun.
- Play is a waste of time if you have better things to do.

The Reality of Play
Play is crucial, creative, and restorative for adults as well as children. It's also more than just having fun, though fun can be a central part of play; it's also about rest, recreation, exploration, and renewal. Play isn't a waste of time because it fosters health benefits through meaningful pleasures, and the emotional benefits of play include development throughout the whole life cycle. These benefits include working out problems, practicing skills, venting tensions, processing and integrating insights, and increasing self-esteem.

Myths About Happiness
- Happiness depends on material well-being.
- Happiness depends on social status and career success.
- Happiness is a result of what you accomplish as an individual.

The Reality of Happiness

In fact, happiness is less linked to circumstances or external events than we tend to think. Our culture proffers materialistic, success-oriented, ego-focused routes to happiness, but the world's great wisdom traditions and current psychological research alike indicate that happiness derives from finding meaning in nonmaterial pleasures, small daily events that prompt satisfaction, engagement with other people, and insights into fundamental truths about life.

To understand more fully how myths affect issues of balance and imbalance, let's look at one of them: the myth of the selfless caretaker. Specifically, let's consider the consequences of one variant of this myth: "To be a good mother, I should always put everyone else in the family ahead of myself."

What's the profile of someone who subscribes to this statement? When we discuss this profile at Structure House, participants make comments like these: "She's overfocused on others' needs"; "She has no time for herself"; "She's probably exhausted." When I ask, "And what does that feel like?" people will answer along these lines: "She's resentful"; "She's angry"; "She's probably depressed"; "She may be feeling unfulfilled." The role of the Good Mother gets a lot of lip service in our culture, but the reality is tough—in fact, it's often a series of ever-escalating goals that society presents. What is the personal impact of this idealization of motherhood? It often takes a significant emotional toll. Participants at Structure House understand the situation, and they say as much: "That kind of superselflessness isn't really doing favors for anybody"; "A person in that role will eventually just burn out"; "She'll wind up feeling really angry that her own needs aren't getting met."

So if these myths complicate rather than simplify the tasks you face in creating balance, how should you respond to them? And how can you creatively address the central dilemma of a need for balance?

Be Structured but Not Rigid

My recommendation is that you approach lifestyle change in much the same way that you approach your eating: become Structured but not rigid. In your wider activities as well as in your food use, Structure provides a sense of order that offers freedom rather than just constraints. To create Structure that fosters balance, I urge you to follow these three steps:

- Look at the time and energy you spend—both in general and in specific aspects of your life (work, relationships, and self-care).
- Assess the satisfaction and meaning you derive from any given aspect.
- Assess how that particular aspect leaves room for other aspects overall—that is, how that aspect may positively or negatively affect other areas of your life.

The big issues are always the same: you need to consider the balance or lack of balance in your life; you need to consider how much a state of imbalance will prompt Unstructured Eating; and you need to explore ways to address issues of imbalance and prevent the toll that it can take.

Ultimately, what I'm asking you to do regarding balance is to reflect on your life's activities as a map. How much of what you see in the layout of your activities is congruent with your deepest values and aspirations? How much of what you do on a day-to-day basis enhances your sense of connectedness to yourself and to others? If examining the actions you take seems balanced and self-sustaining, that's great. If what you see isn't so reassuring—if imbalance in your life leaves you exhausted, stressed, upset, angry, or dissatisfied in other ways—I urge you to look further for ways to balance your life with more meaning, more satisfying activities, and healthy pleasures that provide you with new sources of satisfaction and nurturance.

As you proceed, here are some other aspects of balance to keep in mind:

- Issues of balance shift depending on where you are in the life cycle. Aspects of life that may seem balanced at one stage—such as intense focus on work during the early phase of a career—may seem out of balance at another stage, such as when you're more settled in your work. Your sense of balance or imbalance will change over time.

- Men and women may have different experiences of balance and imbalance. Although these differences are at least partly a consequence of cultural roles and expectations, they are still significant in their ability to affect us all.

- Cultural differences come into play as well, since your cultural background may affect your perception of roles, obligations, relationships, and other issues that affect your sense of balance. Cultural roles and expectations will influence your perceptions of balance or imbalance. Your perceptions of what it means to be "a good parent" or "a high-performing professional," for instance, may exert pressure on your actions, leading to balance or imbalance.

Ultimately, however, your individual needs, wants, capabilities, and goals will have the most influence on whether you feel that your life is balanced or out of balance.

The rest of this chapter will explore two topics related to balance as a way of helping you address these issues.

TASK 2: EXPLORE ACTIVE LEISURE

In our society, we often tend to swing between two extreme attitudes about leisure. One extreme is a tendency toward overwork and an excessive burden of obligations; the other extreme is collapse from fatigue and a reliance on "vegging out" to relieve stress, anxiety, and boredom. Both extremes can prompt a reliance on nonnutritional eating to meet needs for nurturance, stress reduction, pleasure, and entertainment. When I ask Structure House participants why they use food to ease the pressures caused by overwork and heavy responsibility, I hear answers like these: "I'm looking for energy"; "I need stress relief"; It's sort of a safety valve"; or "I'm trying to soothe myself at the end of the day." When I ask about food as a response to boredom, I hear statements like "It helps when I have nothing else to do"; "It fills the gap when nothing else is going on"; and "I need it as an easy way to give myself pleasure."

Reflecting on these situations and the comments they prompt, let's ask a few questions:

- Why is leisure important?
- What prompts so many people to overdo in terms of work and responsibilities and then collapse into passive boredom?
- In what ways does this sort of extremism encourage Unstructured Eating?
- What is the difference between *relaxation* and *collapse*?

It's a myth that relaxation just naturally, automatically happens. On the contrary, relaxation is a structured activity, something you need to prepare for, set conditions for, and defend. It's something you need to make happen. In addition, it's highly personal—something that, ideally, you'll tailor to your own needs and interests. You can't just disengage from the other demands on your attention and instantly attain a relaxed state of mind. How, then, can you achieve relaxation and the creative, replenishing states of leisure that it makes possible?

The Nature of "Optimal Experience"

Mihaly Csikszentmihalyi (pronounced "chick-sent-me-high-ee"), a Hungarian-born American psychologist, has done extensive research on "optimal experience"—the times when people report feelings of concentration and deep enjoyment. Intrigued by how and why people feel these positive states of mind, Csikszentmihalyi studied this seemingly intangible aspect of human experience for several decades. His book *Flow: The Psychology of Optimal Experience* (New York: HarperPerennial, 1990) notes with concern that "[P]eople often end up feeling that their lives have been wasted, that instead of being filled with happiness their years were spent in anxiety and boredom." This observation prompted him to ask two crucial questions: "Is this [anxiety and boredom] because it is the destiny of mankind to remain unfulfilled, each person always wanting more than he or she can have? Or is the pervasive malaise that often sours even our most precious moments the result of our seeking happiness in the wrong places?" Csikszentmihalyi then undertook research to answer these two questions, as well as a third: "When do people feel most happy?"[1]

Detailed interviews with hundreds of people from many different backgrounds provided a fascinating answer. "What I 'discovered,' " wrote Csikszentmihalyi in *Flow,* "was that happiness is not something that *happens.* It is not the result of good fortune or random chance. It is not something that money can buy or power command. It does not depend on outside events, but rather, on how we interpret them. Happiness, in fact, is a condition that must be prepared for, cultivated, and defended privately by each person. People who learn to control inner experience will be able to determine the quality of their lives, which is as close as any of us can come to being happy."

Consider these words for a moment: *Happiness, in fact, is a condition that must be prepared for, cultivated, and defended privately by each person.* Doesn't that sound like Structure? Csikszentmihalyi goes on to say that happiness is characterized by a sense of control, mastery, skill development, concentration, challenge, and complexity. It demands our attention; it requires goal setting and a sense of discipline and practice. Here again we're talking about structured activities. You can't simply expect satisfaction and happiness to *happen;* you need to make decisions about what you want and how you'll attain it. As Csikszentmihalyi summarizes the situation: "To improve life one must improve the quality of experience."

Here's my response to this situation. You've decided to Structure your eating. I urge you to *Structure your life as well*—Structure your activities *specifically and consciously* to give yourself relaxation, pleasure, and happiness. This is a task that requires skills you already possess. I am certain of that. You just haven't applied those skills to this issue yet. It's so important, and the potential benefits are so great, that I want you to stay openminded toward this option.

When was the last time that your mind, your heart, your will, and your body were all in harmony? When was the last time that you felt so involved with something you were doing that you lost track of time? When was the last time that you performed an activity completely for its own enjoyment in the here and now?

Perhaps you have this experience on an ongoing basis. If so, wonderful!

You are lucky indeed. But perhaps you don't have this experience. Perhaps you feel less satisfied—perhaps far less satisfied—with your activities and their effects on your life. If so, read on.

"The Challenges Were in Balance with the Skills"

Here's how Csikszentmihalyi describes his research into optimal experience: "I spoke with chess players, rock climbers, musicians, and inner-city basketball players," he stated in a recent interview, "asking them to describe their experience when what they were doing was really going well." He goes on to state:

> [T]he interviews seemed in many important ways to focus on the same quality of the experience. For instance, the fact that you were completely immersed in what you were doing, that the concentration was very high, that you knew what you had to do moment by moment, that you had very quick and precise feedback as to how well you were doing, and that you felt that your abilities were stretched but not overwhelmed by the opportunities for action. In other words, the challenges were in balance with the skills. And when those conditions were present, you began to forget all the things that bothered you in everyday life, forget the self as an entity separate from what was going on—you felt you were a part of something greater and you were just moving along with the logic of the activity. Everyone said that it was like being carried by a current, spontaneous, effortless, like a flow.

Note what he stated: "the challenges were in balance with the skills." The implication of this statement is central to what we're discussing here. What Csikszentmihalyi calls "flow"—a state of optimal experience—occurs in a middle zone where the challenges you face and the skills you possess are essentially in balance. If your specific skills are too extensive or highly developed for the challenges you face, you'll tend to feel bored. (Suppose you like to play tennis. Imagine playing against a rank newcomer to the sport.) If, on the other hand, your skills are inadequate to meet the challenges you face, you'll tend to feel anxious and stressed. (Imagine playing against Venus or Serena Williams.) So part of what you need to do to attain *active leisure*—and to enter a flow state that is conductive to enjoyment, exhilaration, and happiness—is to find the middle zone in which your skills and the challenges you face are balanced. In that zone, you're more likely to find yourself fully engaged in a process of learning and discovering and growing. Paradoxically, you lose your "self" enough to grow yourself.

Csikszentmihalyi summarizes this state of mind as "being completely involved in an activity for its own sake. The ego falls away. Time flies. Every action, movement, and thought follows inevitably from the previous one, like playing jazz. Your whole being is involved, and you're using your skills to the utmost."

This statement is important in many ways, but one is its implication that the chief barrier to the flow experience is self-consciousness. If you are excessively aware of yourself as you perform an activity, that self-consciousness takes you out of what you're doing and limits your ability to participate in your own actions. This is an issue that I know many overweight people face. Perhaps you've experienced it as well—the tendency to withdraw from activities, to feel inhibited because of heightened self-consciousness, to withdraw further, to feel even more inhibited because your habitual withdrawal leaves you feeling self-conscious . . . In short, there's a vicious cycle that can damage your willingness and your ability to live your own life. This is a painful situation!

So what can you do in response to this dilemma?

Going with the Flow

When people ask me how they can find something enjoyable to do during their leisure time, I often ask them to think about their childhood and the games they played or activities in which they participated. The chances are that similar activities will be fun for them to do in adulthood.

Whether you know it or not, you have undoubtedly experienced flow many times before. You certainly experienced it as a child, because all children routinely enter flow states when playing, exploring the world, and learning—until, unfortunately, they start to unlearn this ability during adolescence. Losing the ability to attain flow is common for many people by the time they reach adulthood. The question now is how to regain it.

Doing so requires setting goals, making choices, and acting on them to develop skills. Here's what I suggest:

- First, determine what you're interested in doing enough to master the necessary skills.

- Second, become *immersed* in the activity—really involved in what you're doing— which requires concentration.

- Third, pay attention to direct experience. This requires sustained involvement— staying engaged, concentrating, developing your skills, being sensitive to feed- back, and overcoming a sense of self-consciousness; paradoxically, growing the self while *losing* yourself in the activity.

Perhaps you'll say, "Well, this sounds great—but what difference does it make, really? Will these activities really do more than just keep me busy?"

Here's a clue. Studies by Salvatore R. Maddi focused on the effects of stress on two thousand people who all reported external stress (deaths in the family, divorce, illness, work stress, and so forth). Within this popula- tion of people experiencing stress, one group seemed more protected from the internal symptoms of stress—depression, anxiety, high blood pressure, overweight, misuse of food, and so forth. The other group had experienced stress, just like the first group, but it didn't manifest the con- sequences. The researchers called this second group "stress hardy." What do you think was the primary distinguishing feature between these groups? It was four to six hours a week of what the researchers called "meaningful activity." For some reason, meaningful activity seemed to provide an element of protection against the effects of life stress.[2]

Four to six hours. That's less than an hour a day. What could that mean for you, to cultivate, defend, and prepare for an activity that would re- quire about an hour of your time each day? This would be your stress management time, your relaxation time.

Another study—this one stemming from work by Csikszentmihalyi and his colleagues—studied flow and optimal experience by giving people pagers to use during their regular daily activity. Throughout the day, the researchers checked with the people being studied, asked them about their activities, and measured their sense of flow, happiness, concentration, and motivation. They would be reading the paper, playing with a child, driving to work, standing in the supermarket, or doing whatever else they were doing. They'd call in, and the researchers would ask, "What are you doing now? How engaged are you in what you're doing? How do you feel?"[3]

What emerged from this research was that the most overall rewarding experience associated with daily activities was in this category of "active leisure." What does this term mean? *Leisure* implies that you're doing what you're doing for it's own sake—because you want to, not because you need to, ought to, or are getting paid to. *Active* means that it's not passive; you're *doing* something yourself, not vicariously experiencing what others are doing, such as by watching actors in a TV show. *Active leisure* means that it's your choice and you're involved in what you're doing. (This definition doesn't rule out having optimal experiences at work. Many people do, in fact, enjoy and get deeply engrossed in their work. But, in general, active leisure usually happens on your own time and on your own turf.) We're talking about pursuing a hobby, exercising, playing sports, playing an instrument, engaging in social activities, and other discretionary activities.

Why do we spend so little time in active versus passive leisure? All too often, what we choose is *passive* leisure. People sit in front of the TV and flip the channels, they surf the Web with nothing much in mind, and they engage in all kinds of other vicarious pastimes. Ironically, these activities usually bring less enjoyment than more active pursuits. Or else they use Unstructured Eating as an "escape hatch" from whatever stress and boredom they're feeling.

What I'm describing may sound like a major logistical challenge. You may protest, "But it's *hard* to do something active!" or "By the end of the day I'm so exhausted that all I want is to kick back."

I understand the situation. Active leisure takes time and effort. It means you have to overcome your sense of caution or self-consciousness. You'll have to experiment with possibilities. You'll have to explore your interests and abilities. All very true. And I know these challenges represent a change from what you may be accustomed to. Still, I believe that accepting the challenges and trying out new possibilities is necessary and, in the long run, will lead to new satisfactions.

For these reasons, I urge you to consider the wealth of opportunities before you. There are many ways to proceed. As a start, I suggest that you look over some or all of the following checklists to consider your options. A good approach to these exercises is to go through the alphabet and come up with an activity for each of the various letters.

Social Interaction Ideas

Alcoholics/Narcotics/Overeaters
  Anonymous
Attend club meetings
Attend parties
Badminton
Baseball
Basketball
Become active in a church
Billiards
Bingo
Board games
Bowling
Ceramics, crafts
Chess/checkers
Church/synagogue study group
Cribbage
Croquet
Darts
Garden clubs
Get involved in a community service
  group
Go dancing
Go to/join a church or synagogue
Golf
Handball
Hockey

Horseshoes
Invite friends to your home
Join a club
Join a political issues group
Junior League
Lawn bowling
Meet/visit with neighbors
Miniature golf
Ping-Pong
Play cards
Racquetball
Reestablish an old friendship
Seek new friends
Skating
Soccer
Softball
Take a class: hobbies, self-improvement
Take a class at a public park or recreation
  area
Take group lessons in athletics: tennis,
  golf, skating
Telephone friends
Volunteer at a hospital
Write letters/e-mail
Other:
Other:

Relaxation Ideas

Bubble bath	Painting
Call a friend	Play an instrument
Daydream	Puzzles
Doodle	Read a novel
Draw	Relaxation techniques
Drink hot tea	Sauna
Get a facial	Singing, humming
Go to a movie	Sunbathe
Hammock	Take a nap
Listen to music	Touch someone you love
Manicure/pedicure	TV
Massage	Walk
Meditation	Yoga
Nature walk	Other:
Needlework	Other:

Spectator Appreciation Ideas That Require Activity

Art galleries	Hockey
Attend plays, musicals, opera	Lawn and garden shows
Ballets	Lectures
Baseball	Museums: history, art, life and science
Basketball	Rodeos
Boat shows	Soccer
Church/synagogue	Special exhibits in your area
Circus	Symphony
Concerts (rock, jazz, blues, etc.)	Talent shows
Craft shows	Tennis
Daydreaming by a lake or river	Travel
Football	Volleyball
Go sightseeing	Watch movies at a theater
Golf	Zoo
Gymnastics	Other:
Historical sites	Other:

Physical Exercise Ideas

Aerobic dance

Avoid elevators

Backpacking

Badminton

Baseball

Basketball

Bicycling

Bowling

Canoeing

Dancing

Fencing

Fitness courses

Football

Frisbee golf

Gardening

Golf—if you walk

Gymnastics

Handball

Hiking

Hockey

Home repair

Horseback riding

Ice skating

Jogging

Judo

Karate

Lacrosse

Landscaping

Lot softball

Racquetball

Rock climbing

Roller skating

Rugby

Sailing

Scuba diving

Sex

Shelling

Sky diving

Snorkeling

Snow skiing

Soccer

Squash

Swimming

T'ai chi

Tennis

Volleyball

Volunteer work

Walking

Water aerobics

Water flex and tone

Waterskiing

Water volleyball

Weight lifting

Wind surfing

Wood refinishing

Other: ·

Other:

Intellectual Stimulation Ideas

Anagrams

Backgammon

Boggle

Brain teasers

Cards

Checkers

Chess

Computer

Creative writing

Crossword puzzles

Discuss current events/controversial
   subjects

Documentaries

Dominoes

Go to museums

Jigsaw puzzles

Join a debate club

Journal writing

Lectures

Letter writing

Library

Magazines/newspapers

Meditation

Reading

Reading poetry

Scrabble

Seminars

Stock market

Take a class in something you'd like

Take a self-improvement class

Travel

Trivial Pursuit

Video games

Visit historical sites

Worship services

Writing poetry

Other:

Other:

Creative Expression Ideas

Acting/drama club/skits

Calligraphy

Candle making

Car restoration

Ceramics

Composing

Crafts

Creative writing

Crocheting/knitting

Dance

Découpage

Drawing

Gardening

Interior decorating

Journal writing

Landscaping

Leatherwork

Macramé

Metalwork

Model building

Needlework

Painting

Photography

Playing an instrument

Pottery

Puppetry

Quilting

Rug hooking

Sculpture

Sewing

Singing

Stained-glass work

Stenciling

Storytelling

Upholstering

Weaving

Wood refinishing/Woodworking

Other:

These lists are obviously just a starting point. To benefit from active leisure, you have to sort through your options, try out some possibilities, and see what happens. Perhaps you'll find something that interests you right off. Perhaps you'll have to try out all kinds of options before you find what suits you. There are no guarantees. Given the potential for change and growth, though, it's worthwhile to start.

TASK 3: EXPLORE THE OPTIONS FOR HEALTHY PLEASURES

Western medical science has generally focused on studying problems and disease. Up until recently, Western psychology, too, has concerned itself primarily with pathology—mental illness, dysfunction, and abnormal behavior. The emphases have, in short, been the negative aspects of human existence. In recent decades, however, researchers have turned their attention to more positive experiences—a shift that raised some intriguing questions.

- What is the nature of happiness, and how can we increase our options for attaining it?
- Is happiness a fundamental state, or is it the result of numerous, small experiences that add up over time?
- How can we enrich our lives and move more consistently in the direction of growth?
- In what ways can we see health not just as the absence of disease and dysfunction but also as a positive force in its own right?

The answers to these questions are incomplete; however, the efforts to understand them have already led to indications that positive experience, pleasure, and a sense of meaning have direct benefits for our health. In addition, recent studies suggest specific ways of increasing satisfaction with daily life.

Throughout this book, we've discussed the importance of looking at your relationship to food. Understanding this relationship can have tangible benefits as you address issues of overweight and health. In many ways, however, what you're really looking at is your relationship to life in general—the quality of your life, your level of engagement with the world, and the depth of satisfaction, meaning, and pleasure that you feel. Ask yourself these important questions:

- Once you've put a healthy, structured diet into place, how can you allow yourself to experience the natural pleasures available to you through *all* of your senses?

- How can you learn to focus on the richness of your own experience at any given moment?

- What's the difference between *what you're experiencing* and *your assessment (or judgment) of what you're experiencing?*

- To live fully and openly in response to your own full experience of life, can you create a plan for meaningful pleasures in your life—what we could call a "minimum daily requirement" of pleasure? Are you willing to experiment with new kinds of healthy pleasures to help you attain this goal?

The Question of Happiness

These questions presents us with a basic and age-old question: What is happiness? We aren't going to answer this question—one that philosophers, poets, theologians, psychologists, and countless others have wrestled with through the ages—but I believe it's important at least to ask it.

Some of the possibilities are fairly straightforward. As the psychologist Abraham Maslow has described in his writings about what he calls the "hierarchy of needs," happiness is partly a result of having your physical and emotional needs met. It's partly a result of not being in a state of inner or outer conflict. But what else accounts for happiness? There's reason to believe that once a person's needs are met, happiness ultimately isn't derived from external elements—possessions, accomplishments, status, power. In fact, various kinds of psychological research indicate that satisfaction and happiness are largely results of a person's ability to connect more deeply *with his or her experience of living*—with the small and often subtle events and pleasures that make up daily life.

One of the interesting implications of recent research is that major life events—positive and negative alike—have relatively little effect on people's long-term happiness. Robert Ornstein and David Sobel, in their book *Healthy Pleasures,* provide these two examples: one person wins the lottery, and another person suffers a severe accident and becomes paraplegic. I'm sure we'd all label the first event "positive" and the second one "negative." Yet Ornstein and Sobel's research shows that even winning the lottery or suffering a disabling accident are events that tend *not* to alter people's fundamental happiness or lack of happiness. Both events would, of course, have an initial impact. But after a certain period—roughly a year—people tend to "reset" and go back to their original level of happiness.[4]

There's also been research showing that marriage doesn't necessarily change a person's degree of happiness to a significant degree. This outcome flies in the face of cultural expectations that getting married is transformative: if you're unhappy, just go to the chapel, say "I do," and all will be well. In fact, someone who expects marriage to shift his or her happiness on a daily basis will probably find that at least in the long term, happiness eventually "resets" to wherever it was before the wedding.

So if major, life-changing events aren't what determine happiness and unhappiness, what does? Researchers into this subject suggests that happiness has four key components:

- **Pleasure:** enjoying what you're doing in the present moment
- **Engagement:** feeling deeply involved in what you're doing
- **Satisfaction and meaning:** using your personal strengths to serve some larger end
- **Quality of experience and connection:** feeling a sense of relationship to yourself, to other people, to other beings, to life, to activities, and to your own experience

Take Steps Toward a More Satisfying Life

Sonja Lyubomirsky, a psychologist at the University of California who specializes in research about happiness, has compiled a list of steps people can take to increase satisfaction in their lives. Some of these steps are designed to provide a temporary mood boost; others are entry points to pursuing greater satisfaction, engagement, and meaning. Here are Lyubomirsky's suggested steps:[5]

- **Count your blessings.** Keep a "gratitude journal" of events that prompt you to feel grateful. These can range from the mundane (your flowers bloom) to the magnificent (your child takes her first steps).

- **Practice and cultivate kindness.** Kind acts should be both random (letting a harried mom go ahead of you at the supermarket checkout line) and systematic (taking supper to an elderly neighbor).

- **Savor life's joys.** Taste the sweetness of a strawberry and feel the warmth of the sun. Tune in to the present moment even when you're in the middle of a difficult experience.

- **Thank a mentor.** Write a letter of thanks to someone who guided you or taught you—or thank him or her in person.

- **Learn to forgive.** Write a letter of forgiveness to someone who hurt or wronged you, as doing so will help to free you from obsessive rumination and allow you to move on.

- **Invest time and energy in friends and family.** One of the most potent sources of happiness is strong personal relationships.

- **Take care of your body.** By getting enough sleep and exercise, and by smiling and laughing, you can boost your mood in the short term and contribute to your deeper satisfaction in the long term.

- **Develop strategies for coping with stress and hardships.** Make meaning out of difficulties, and choose growth and wisdom in the face of life's pain.

Find Pleasure Channels

My hope is that as you've read this book, you've realized that a major part of coping with overweight and health issues involves changing your relationship with food. I want you to look at the bigger picture as well. If food has been functioning as a stress reducer, as a way of easing loneliness, or as a way of compensating for a lack of meaning or engagement with the world, I want you to open your mind to other options. I want you to consider relationships, activities, and sensual pleasures that more fully support your deeper health goals. Let's look at positive indulgences that have the greatest chance of fostering a sense of engagement and meaning. By their very nature, children know how to derive pleasure from life. Kids' playfulness and ability to live "in the moment" appear to be biologically determined. A capacity for pleasure and enjoyment is in our DNA; we are programmed to desire enjoyment as part of survival. Numerous studies show that positive experiences—whether laughter or spending time with a loved one—boost your immunity and provide other health benefits. Unfortunately, most adults have lost their earlier capacity for spontaneous enjoyment of life. But that capacity can be rediscovered and revitalized— something I strongly recommend. Four important questions to ask:

- What are some activities for which you might want to give yourself positive indulgences and tap into pleasure in a healthier way?
- What is your prescription for incorporating more healthy pleasures into your lifestyle?
- What is your "minimum daily requirement" of pleasure?
- How are you going to build in healthy pleasures on a daily basis for your plan?

My recommendation is what Ornstein and Sobel term *pleasure channels*. These are the various ways in which we allow pleasurable experiences into our lives. The goal: to nourish yourself with a rich, healthy feast of sensory experiences and to set aside judgmental states of mind and mental "filters" that prevent you from experiencing life freshly and directly. Rather than resorting to Unstructured Eating as a habitual, counterproductive approach, use a wider range of pleasures to provide delight, relief, and stimulation in your life.

Design a Recreational Program

There are six ingredients in a well-balanced recreational program: social interaction, creative expression, physical exercise, spectator appreciation, intellectual stimulation, and solitary relaxation. Everyone needs all of these to some degree. However, different people fulfill different needs in different recreational pursuits. The following charts represent a very small fraction of activities available to help you meet the need for a well-balanced, personal recreation program. These activities are, however, some of the most commonly utilized by a majority of persons between the ages of 20 and 65. In any case, this survey is merely a starting point for looking into your own strengths and weaknesses in these recreational areas.

Here is how to score your results. Place a check mark in the appropriate indulgence column. Score 3 points for "frequently," 2 points for "occasionally," and 1 point for "never." Add up each section. A score of 18 to 23 is considered normal for each individual section. Then add up all the section totals to arrive at the overall picture. The scoring for the total is at the end.

Social Interaction	Frequently	Occasionally	Never
I invite friends to visit my home.			
I seek new friends.			
I write letters/e-mail.			
I attend parties.			
I play cards.			
I visit neighbors.			
I attend club meetings.			
I socialize during activities.			
I spend time with friends/family.			
I telephone friends.			

Social Interaction total: _____

Creative Expression	Frequently	Occasionally	Never
I cook low-cal gourmet food.			
I plan parties.			
I plan landscapes/gardens.			
I do handicrafts/woodworking.			
I write poetry or stories.			
I compose music or sing.			
I paint or draw pictures.			
I plan/do home redecoration.			
I do photography.			
I participate in theater/drama/dance.			

Creative Expression total: _____

Physical Exercise	Frequently	Occasionally	Never
I work in the garden or yard.			
I take walks.			
I avoid taking the elevator.			
I dance.			
I ride a bicycle.			
I refinish antiques.			
I fish, hunt, or camp.			
I pick wildflowers.			
I wash the car.			
I take part in active sports.			

Physical Exercise total: _____

Spectator Appreciation	Frequently	Occasionally	Never
I watch television.			
I attend movies.			
I go to athletic/cultural events.			
I watch children at play.			
I notice changes in buildings and landscapes.			
I bird-watch.			
I travel or go sightseeing.			
I people-watch.			
I see stage plays/musicals.			
I attend concerts.			

Spectator Appreciation total: _____

Intellectual Stimulation	Frequently	Occasionally	Never
I attend lectures.			
I actively participate in service to others.			
I visit the art museum.			
I discuss controversial subjects.			
I go to the library.			
I collect something.			
I keep up on current events.			
I take time to answer questions from kids.			
I watch documentaries.			
I read newspapers/magazines/nonfiction.			

Intellectual Stimulation total: _____

Solitary Relaxation	Frequently	Occasionally	Never
I read.			
I work crossword or jigsaw puzzles.			
I hum, whistle, or sing to myself.			
I listen to tapes/CDs.			
I keep a scrapbook.			
I sit on the porch by myself.			
I take relaxing baths.			
I daydream/take naps.			
I watch snow fall/listen to rain.			
I do prayer/meditation.			

Solitary Relaxation Total: _____

Overall Leisure Total: _____

Total Score

Under 80	Are you sure you're alive? Check your pulse.
81–100	That old rockin' chair is yours.
101–139	You have a well-balanced recreational program.
140–160	You have an extraordinary zest for life—or else you can't add!
161–180	It's a wonder you can keep up with yourself. Slow down!

Wake Up Your Senses as a Healthy Way to Stimulate, Inspire, and Soothe Yourself[6]

We live in a culture that encourages distraction. TV, radio, computers, and other gadgets bombard us constantly—and numb us, lull us, agitate us, and hijack us out of the present moment of our own experience. One effect of this situation is that our senses end up overwhelmed and blunted. We are simultaneously overstimulated and dissatisfied.

How can you reconnect with your senses? How can you begin to reconnect with sensory experience on a daily basis in ways that enable you to be more fully present in the enjoyment of daily life? How can you take better care of your body and mind?

Let's look at each of the senses and explore them as healthy ways to soothe, stimulate, inspire, enliven, and reassure yourself.

Wake Up Your Sense of Vision

Have you noticed how dogs, cats, and many other animals often simply gaze at the world around them? Have you ever watched young children stare at the sights they see? As adults, we often forget to notice what's before us, much less *observe* anything with close, focused attention. Give yourself a vibrant, rich, nourishing feast through the sense of sight.

Buy a beautiful flower or plant; make a space in a room delightful; light a candle and watch the flame. Set a pretty place at the table, using your best dishes and silverware. Go to a museum and contemplate the art. Go sit in the lobby of an attractive old hotel. Closely observe nature around you. Go out in the middle of the night and watch the stars. Gaze at a landscape at dawn, at sunset, or in bright moonlight. Observe the architecture in a historic part of town. Shape your nails so they look nice. Look at interesting photography in a book. Go to a dance performance or a sporting event. Watch people as you sit at a sidewalk café. Take the time to observe your surroundings closely, taking in the light and the colors, allowing yourself to gaze fully and deeply. Be mindful of each sight that passes before you.

Wake Up Your Sense of Hearing

Do you feel different when you listen to reggae as compared to Gregorian chant? The Beatles as compared to techno rock? How do the sounds of nature, of church bells, of children laughing all affect you? Sounds change and shape your moods. Tap into that and celebrate the power of hearing. Give yourself a mood transplant with sound.

Listen to inspiring or soothing music or to invigorating and exciting music. Pay attention to the sounds of nature (waves, birds, rainfall, leaves rustling, silence). Sing or whistle to your favorite song. Hum a soothing tune. Sing in a chorus. Learn to play an instrument. Pound on a drum—or a tabletop. Listen to books on tape. Call an information number to observe a human voice. Clink a spoon against a wineglass. Record and play back your voice reading a poem or a letter. Be mindful of any sounds that come your way, letting them go in one ear and out the other, just noticing the rise and fall of vibrations and the space between sounds.

Wake Up Your Sense of Touch

Touch is soothing; touch is stimulating. As human beings, we are highly tactile creatures, yet we often live in ways that are touch-deprived. This state can create a kind of "skin hunger"—a craving for touching and being touched.

Take a hot bubble bath. Put clean sheets on your bed. Pet your dog or cat. Have a massage. Soak your feet. Put creamy lotion on your whole body. Put a cold compress on your forehead or a heating pad on your lower back. Sink into a really comfortable chair in your home, or find one in a luxurious hotel lobby. Put on a silky blouse, robe, or scarf. Notice the sensations of clothing on your body. Try on cashmere gloves in a department store. Brush your hair for a long time or massage your scalp gently. Hug someone and pause before letting go. Allow yourself to experience whatever you are touching.

Wake Up Your Sense of Taste

We often eat in rushed, mechanical ways that limit our ability to taste what we eat, or else we use food to "numb out" in ways that don't offer much pleasure. My recommendation: pay attention to the experiences of textures, flavors, and subtle aspects of food that make the sense of taste such a rich experience.

Really taste a good meal. Have a favorite soothing drink, such as herbal tea or decaf coffee. Get a little bit of a special food you don't usually spend the money on, such as fresh herbs. Allow your attention to taste the food you eat fully and savor each slow bite; eat the meal mindfully. When you find yourself distracted by thoughts or emotions, gently bring your attention back to the tastes and textures in your mouth.

Wake Up Your Sense of Smell

We live in a world that's rich with scents and aromas. Think of how different your yard smells following a rainstorm than when it's dry. Consider how different the land smells in winter, spring, summer, and fall. Notice all the varied scents as you walk through a garden in full bloom. Imagine how impoverished we'd be if we lacked a sense of smell.

Use your favorite cologne or lotion, or try out some new scent in a store. Spray fragrance in the air. Light a scented candle. Put lemon oil on your furniture. Put potpourri in a bowl in your room. Boil cinnamon sticks. Smell the roses. Notice the scent of a pet's fur or a baby's skin. Breathe in the aromas of a nutritious meal or a cup of hot tea before you begin and while you're eating or drinking. Walk in a wooded area and mindfully breathe in the fresh smells of nature.

Wake Up Your Sense of Movement

In addition to what we call the five senses, we humans also have *proprioception*, a neuromuscular response to how we perceive our bodies in motion. Moving feels good and can stimulate feelings of delight and well-being. Can you build creative movement into your lifestyle? I have learned over the years that people who are overweight or obese don't have a sense of their bodies in space or in motion.

Take a dance class—or go dancing with friends. If you're too shy, put on music at home and dance right then and there. Take a yoga class. Study t'ai chi. Learn about mindful walking. Take a brisk walk in the park. Go swimming. Ride a bike. Play on the grass with a child.

Wake Up Your Brain

We don't usually think of the mind as a sensory organ, but it's not just a computer—a thinking machine. There's more and more evidence that the brain is fully involved in active awareness, not just passive processing of information. People who walk every day show better cognition and protection against Alzheimer's disease. Those who exercise the brain do much better in coping in life overall.

Read a challenging book. Speak with someone who stimulates your thinking. Join a debating society. Take a writing workshop. Learn a new language. Take a class in a subject you know nothing about. Buy a book of puzzles and mind-teasers. Watch instructional videos. Learn a new skill—cooking, woodworking, flower arranging, or whatever else interests you.

Wake Up Your Intuition

There's something within you that's capable of deep insight—gut-level hunches or "felt knowledge" about people, events, and choices. Maybe you call it your heart space, your inner wisdom, or your spirit. What is that—and how can you gain better access to it, validate it, and cultivate it?

Practice contemplation or meditation. Write in a journal. Start psychotherapy with a thoughtful psychologist, counselor, or social worker. Take a yoga class. Read books about philosophy or theology. Read the wisdom literature and holy books of Judaism, Christianity, and the other great religions. Pray, either alone or in a group. Find other sources of spiritual insight, deep happiness, and transcendent meaning.

I want to revisit and amplify some questions I asked at the start of this chapter.

However many years you live, what will your life ultimately mean? What will those years be about? How will you see your place on Earth during that time? Will you see your life as a work of art—or as a formless blur? What will your sense be of what has taken place? Will your life seem like something in which you've actively participated? Or will it be something that has simply occurred and passed you by?

Part of lifestyle change is validating and incorporating healthy pleasures into your life rather than denying, dismissing, diminishing them. This process is crucial in its own right; it's how you stay open to life's richness and continue developing over the years.

Part of lifestyle change is also challenging yourself: trying out new experiences even when they seem unfamiliar and daunting. Celebrate partial successes even if you're striving for a preconceived notion of success. Try to understand what's working and what isn't. Give yourself room to grow.

Finally, I urge you to see what I'm describing as an ongoing process, not as a short-term event. Don't judge yourself or spend time on self-critical attitudes. Accept your own creativity and wisdom regarding what you need to do. You probably know what you need. Now be curious, explore, and be open to yourself. By trusting your own insights, you can become more skillful, more alert, more aware.

Conclusion:
Take the Journey

At the start of *The Structure House Weight Loss Plan*, I stated that this is a book about change. I also stated that the change I was referring to is more important than the kind of change you can measure by stepping on your bathroom scale. Weight loss matters, of course, but it's not what matters most. Changing your perceptions of yourself, changing your relationship with food, and changing your choices about how to live are all more significant than changing the number on the dial.

The discussions in this book are intended to help you feel more open toward change, accepting the possibility of change and the benefits of change, which will give you many new options.

At the same time, I'm aware that change can be daunting. Change means leaving behind what's familiar. Change means moving ahead into unknown territory. Change means accepting that you can be different from what you are now. These options may be exciting, but they are also potentially demanding—demanding of insights, demanding of effort, demanding of flexibility. But it's no reason to shy away from change.

Here's the truth about change. It's not as hard as you imagine. It doesn't require overnight transformation, only a willingness to consider new ideas little by little over the long term. It doesn't require perfection, only a willingness to persist in trying out new behaviors with some consistency and patience. In fact, changing even a few key behaviors can be so life-enhancing, so empowering, and so enjoyable that the process of change can develop a powerful momentum of its own. Change brings joy. Change can also bring a cycle of positive consequence—the opposite of the vicious cycle I described earlier—and this cycle of positive consequences can become self-perpetuating. Changed behavior leads to good feelings about yourself, which lead in turn to more changed behaviors, which lead to less reliance on food, which leads to good feelings about yourself, and so on, around and around.

It's hard for me to summarize the Structure House program and offer you a tidy end point to our many varied discussions. Perhaps the simplest way for me to conclude is to emphasize that what I've been advocating throughout this book is a journey. Each person who uses the Structure House program embarks on a journey of change. This journey is a process; it has stages; and it evolves over time. Like many journeys, this one may seem different from what you expected when you first set out. The journey may also take you to a destination that's different—more interesting, more remarkable—than the one you envisioned at the start. More challenging? Maybe so; maybe not.

Here's a series of comments that will provide both a backward glance at what we've discussed and a look ahead to the journey I urge you to undertake. The first set of comments under each topic is mine. Then I quote some recent Structure House participants—each of them a Student of Change who is making this same journey.

THE JOURNEY STARTS BY TAKING RESPONSIBILITY

Your journey will begin when you feel discomfort, even outright pain. Why then? Because if you're comfortable, you want to stay where you are; if you feel discomfort, you want to change your situation. It's human nature for you to seek a different place, a better place, if you feel restless, unhappy, burdened, or pained. That's why the change we're talking about often requires that you focus on the negative—on what isn't working, on what feels unpleasant, on what prompts dissatisfaction. This is your inspiration to do something different. Reread your "Dear Me" letter. Is this how you want to live? Is this what you want to be?

Now take responsibility for your state of being. Choose to change. Make a plan. Get ready to take the first steps.

> "We're adults, no one's going to fix us, we're not victims. We may have been [victims] as children . . . but we're no longer victims. There *is* a solution. There is hope."
>
> —Peter

> "You have to make yourself accountable—that's the only way to lose the weight and keep it off. Accountability comes down to the Food Diary and self-honesty. You can lie in the diary really fast. Weigh yourself. Measurements are also a way to be accountable."
>
> —Sallie

WEIGHT LOSS ALONE ISN'T THE DESTINATION

Millions of people lose weight but then regain the pounds, sometimes repeating this cycle of lose/gain/lose/gain over and over. If you mistakenly view weight loss as the end of the journey ("All I need to do is lose weight"), you won't succeed in the long run. But if you can view weight loss as something that happens during the first half of the journey, you can view the rest of the journey as a more gradual process of lifestyle change, self-understanding, and growth. If you can understand this approach and dedicate yourself to it, you're much more likely to succeed. You will have become a Student of Change.

> "Everybody can go to a bookstore and buy any book . . . about diet and eat 1,800 calories, no more than 25 percent of calories from fat. We all know how to do it. We can all be programmed for a while as robots and do it. . . . The

problem is the day after. . . . If you go back to the same environment as you came from . . . nothing [has] changed."

—Aaron

FAD DIETS AREN'T THE RIGHT PATH

Fad diets focus on something external to you. They never address the *un-derlying imbalances* that make you vulnerable to using food. By accepting responsibility for change and seeking the skills that facilitate change, you can develop a healthier relationship with food and thus address the issues that will make deeper, longer-lasting change possible.

"I think we all know on some level there's no shortcut. And all these fad diets only work in the short term."

—Peter

"Everyone is looking for a quick fix today, but there's no silver bullet."

—Jack

IT'S NOT *FOOD* THAT MAKES YOU FAT

What do I mean by "underlying imbalances"? It's the use of food in ways that go beyond nutrition. As I often tell Structure House participants, "Nobody comes here for a weight problem." *Weight is only a symptom of an underlying imbalance in your relationship with food.* When your relation-ship with food gets out of balance, you use food in nonnutritional ways, and then you begin to gain weight.

"You have the ability to recognize that you've got a prob-lem and that you're in denial. It's very simple: We're fat because we eat too much and exercise too little. We're not able to eat unstructured without consequences. If you're committed to losing weight, the program will work. It's like everything else: *interest* doesn't cut it; it's *commitment* that makes it happen."

—Jack

"Don't focus on the numbers, focus on your behavior."

—Anella

BALANCE AND IMBALANCE ARE CRUCIAL ISSUES

Many Structure House participants say, "My life is out of balance." These imbalances make people vulnerable to Unstructured Eating, which can lead to weight gain, health problems, and a tendency toward social isolation. If you address your nutritional issues but ignore the wider issues of balance and imbalance, you're unlikely to change your life in ways that matter most.

"Balance is the key."

—Peter

"Remember who you are—do not let your urge to eat identify and control you."

—Kate

STRUCTURE IS A PROBLEM-SOLVING STRATEGY

Structure is a system designed to isolate unhealthy eating, to identify and then address the reasons it occurs, to illuminate how we use food in our lives, to shine a spotlight on our relationship with food, and to show us where we need to make changes.

"Structure is a freedom. It felt like it was a control, but it's a freedom."

—Peter

"The classes [at Structure House] were talking about what goes on in your head—the situations that trigger the eating. Maybe it's that you're not in control, or that you're sad, or whatever. How do I identify these things? How can I be productive rather than being destructive by using food?"

—Lisa

THE KEY TO PROGRESS ON THE JOURNEY: ANTECEDENTS

If the Structure House approach is a journey, the key to progress on this journey is understanding *antecedents*, or "eating triggers." Understanding why you resort to Unstructured Eating is the way you'll understand which behaviors you need to change. Steady progress is easier and more reliable if you monitor yourself through the Structure House Diary—including a record of your activities, your eating, and your weight.

"The food diary is very helpful. It's wonderful. When you're tracking in the food diary you see results."

—Anella

"I found the diary crucial. When I don't write in it, things go steadily downhill."

—Sandra

"If you're eating more than your three meals a day, you need to stop and ask why. What am I looking for? What effect am I looking for? I know now."

—Jack

"Like I'll go, 'I'm really tired today,' or 'I'm really angry today,' or 'Wow, I feel really great today.' I'll see a pattern, and I'll say, 'Oh, I was really great, and then I wore myself down.' Well, that tells you something, doesn't it?"

—Peter

THE JOURNEY IS A PROCESS, NOT A ONE-SHOT EVENT

To make the journey does not require perfection. Only commitment is necessary. Everyone gets Unstructured some of the time, and that's fine. When Unstructured Eating happens, it becomes a learning experience. Using the Diary helps you learn about the circumstances that prompt your Unstructured Eating. The insights this creates will teach you what to change and how to change. As a student of change, you can redefine your relationship with food.

It's important to break this process down into baby steps. One day a participant said to me in despair, "I have 170 pounds to lose! I don't even know where to begin." I told her, "You don't have 170 pounds to lose. You have *one* pound to lose. Just think about losing that one pound first. Then go ahead and lose the next pound." We all have a tendency to look only at the final goal rather than taking things one a day at a time. When you break the task down like that, anyone can do it.

> "I do like quantifiable results and have set up a little point system for myself. I measure positives instead of negatives. I give myself points for going to the gym, for drinking water, for planning meals and sticking to my plan, for tracking my antecedents, for taking care of myself. It's completely changed the way I view the problem."
>
> —Anella

> "Reward yourself for small accomplishments. Set small goals and reward yourself when you succeed. Keep a record of those accomplishments so you can look back and say, 'I really have made progress.' "
>
> —Sallie

STRUCTURE IS A LIFELONG COMMITMENT

Overweight is a chronic problem. Once you develop it, you have to deal with it for the long term. This doesn't mean Structure for a week, two weeks, four weeks, or two months. It's not even for the period during which you lose your weight. Structure is a commitment you make for the long term.

But rest easy. After a while, what you'll do isn't that difficult. You're doing it already in some form or other. Think of the Structure House Diary. Some people say, "Oh, my gosh, a diary!" But in reality, they're probably keeping a day planner or some other form of annotated schedule. The Structure House Diary is no different. It's just a method for keeping your commitment to the journey—how you plan the route you're taking, how you note your progress.

> "When you get to a weight you want, you're going to do the same things you've been doing. That isn't going to change. You'll eat three meals a day, with no snacks. You're going to exercise. You're going to plan your meals. You'll be practicing the whole time."
>
> —Lisa

"FAILURE" IS NEVER FAILURE

When you become Unstructured—which happens to everyone—there's a tendency to think that all is lost. A Structure House participant once berated himself as we spoke because, as he put it, "I've been totally Unstructured."

I asked what had happened.

"I ate a piece of pie."

So I asked him, "How long did it take to eat that piece of pie?"

"Oh, about five minutes."

This intrigued me. "So what did you do the rest of the day? What else did you eat?"

"I didn't eat anything else that I shouldn't have," he replied. "I was Structured."

"Let me get this straight. There are twenty-four hours in the day and sixty minutes in each hour. That makes one thousand four hundred forty minutes in the day. You were Structured for all of that time except for just five minutes?"

"Right."

"For one thousand four hundred thirty-five minutes that day you were Structured, and for five minutes you were Unstructured, but you say you've been Unstructured the whole time?"

"Well . . ."

He got the point.

My recommendation to him—and you—is to develop a different mind-set. Don't regard the normal ups and downs of the journey as "failure."

> "Don't be discouraged by setbacks. Everyone has them. You can always turn it around at any moment."
>
> —Anella

THE JOURNEY ISN'T JUST YOUR PROGRESS; IT'S ALSO THE TOOLS YOU USE

We all take tools on a car trip: a spare tire, a jack, a set of wrenches. You'll need skills on your journey, too—"tools" for the toolbox you'll take along for the ride. What will you take that's useful? How about the Structure House Diary—a way of structuring your activities and your meals ahead of time. How about exercise . . . How about weighing yourself every day . . . How about a support system of some kind—or several kinds—whether that means a group support (Overeaters Anonymous, Weight Watchers) or individual psychotherapy . . . How about nutritional advice . . . How about good exercise advice . . . There are so many specific tools you can acquire and use to make the journey easier!

"Use the diary. Write things down. If you're gaining a whole bunch of weight and are baffled, look at your diary. The answer is usually pretty obvious."

—Anella

"It's a skill. It's a lifelong commitment. It takes effort. You have to be Structured. You have to pay attention to what you're doing. You're learning a skill that you've never had before in your life. But to gain that skill, you have to practice, practice, practice."

—Arthur

"You have to have a support system—whether that support system is e-mail, a therapist, a friend who's willing to listen, a support group of overeaters, or a combination of all of the above. Don't isolate yourself to just one thing."

—Sallie

This is a journey worth taking. It's true that you can't truly understand the destination beforehand, but that's part of what makes moving forward worthwhile and exciting. What you know is that you aren't happy where you are now. This is the starting point. The big question you face is whether to accept the status quo or explore the alternatives.

What is painful in your life?

What isn't working well in your life?

What would you like to be different in your life?

Wouldn't it be wonderful to explore what your life can become?

With courage and some new ideas, you can make the journey toward change.

Appendix 1

Understanding Your Body Mass Index

Your body mass index (BMI) is a number calculated from your weight and height. Although BMI does not measure body fat directly, research has shown that BMI is a reliable indicator of body fatness for people, and it correlates to more high-tech measures of body fat, such as underwater weighing and dual energy X-ray absorptiometry (DXA). BMI has the added advantage of being inexpensive and easy to perform. Your BMI can help your physician identify possible weight problems.[1]

HOW CAN YOU CALCULATE YOUR BMI?

If you want to calculate your own BMI, use one of the following formulas.

Metric System

The formula for BMI is weight in kilograms divided by height in meters squared. Since height is commonly measured in centimeters, divide height in centimeters by 100 to obtain height in meters:

BMI = weight ÷ height^2
Example: weight = 68 kg, height = 165 cm (1.65 m)
Calculation: 68 ÷ 2.7225 = 24.98

Pounds and Inches

To calculate BMI using pounds and inches, you divide your weight in pounds by height in inches squared, then multiply by a conversion factor of 703.

BMI = weight ÷ height^2 × 703
Example: weight = 150 lbs, height = 5'5" (65")
Calculation: [150 ÷ 4225] × 703 = 24.96

WHAT IF I DON'T WANT TO DO THE MATH?

If you want to use an easy calculator to determine your BMI, go to the Web site for the Centers for Disease Control, which provides an online calculator at:

www.cdc.gov/nccdphp/dnpa/bmi/adult_BMI/english_bmi_calculator/bmi_calculator.htm

HOW DO I INTERPRET MY BMI?

For adults 20 and older, you interpret the results of your BMI calculations by using standard weight status categories that are the same for all ages and for both men and women. (Note: calculating and interpreting BMI results for children and teens is a different process. If you need information and guidance about calculations for someone under the age of 20, visit the Centers for Disease Control at http://apps.nccd.cdc.gov/dnpabmi/Calculator.aspx.)

The standard weight status categories associated with BMI ranges for adults are shown below.

Below 18.5: Underweight
18.5 to 24.9: Normal
25.0 to 29.9: Overweight
30.0 and above: Obese

Appendix 2

Understanding Metabolism

To lose weight safely and effectively, you need to know how many calories you can consume. Knowing that figure shouldn't be guesswork; there's a straightforward formula you can use to find out the answer.

WHAT IS YOUR RESTING METABOLIC RATE (RMR)?

The resting metabolic rate is the number of calories needed to sustain the body at rest. Using what's called the Mifflin–St. Jeor equation,[1] here's how you calculate your RMR. (A hint to math-shy readers: what follows is really quite straightforward and easy. Just use a calculator, punch in the numbers, and follow the steps.)

Step 1. _____ ÷ 2.21 = _____
          weight in pounds   result for step 1
                                        (weight in kilograms)

Step 2. _____ × 2.54 = _____
          height in inches   result for step 2
                                        (height in centimeters)

Step 3. $10 \times$ _____ = _____

              result from step 1   result for step 3

              (weight in kilograms)

Step 4. $6.25 \times$ _____ = _____

              result from step 2   result for step 4

              (height in centimeters)

Step 5. $5 \times$ _____ = _____

              age in years   result for step 5

Step 6.
Women:

RMR = _____ + _____ − _____ − 161 = _____

    result from step 3   result from step 4   result from step 5   RMR

Men:

RMR = _____ + _____ − _____ + 5 = _____

    result from step 3   result from step 4   result from step 5   RMR

Total Number of Calories Needed to Maintain Present Weight

It's important to take exercise into account, so select your level of activity and the activity factor below it.

- If you are sedentary (little or no exercise):
  RMR $\times$ 1.2 = total number of calories to maintain weight

- If you are lightly active (exercise 1 to 3 hours per week):
  RMR $\times$ 1.3 = total number of calories to maintain weight

- If you are moderately active (exercise 3 to 5 hours per week):
  RMR $\times$ 1.4 = total number of calories to maintain weight

- If you are very active (exercise 6 to 7 hours per week):
  RMR $\times$ 1.5 = total number of calories to maintain weight

Step 7. _____ $\times$ _____ = _____
　　　　　　RMR　　　　　　　　　activity factor　　　　　　result from step 7
　　　　　　　　　　　　　　　　　　　　　　　　　　　　　　　　calories to
　　　　　　　　　　　　　　　　　　　　　　　　　　maintain present weight

Minimum Number of Calories Needed to Lose Weight at a Healthy Rate (1 percent of Weight per Week)

Finally, follow these last few steps to identify your ideal minimum number of calories per day:

Step 8. _____ $\times$ 0.01 = _____
　　　　　　　　present weight　　　　　　　　　　　1 percent of present weight

Step 9. _____ $\times$ 500 = _____
　　　　　1 percent of present weight　　　　　　　　　result for step 9

Step 10. _____ $-$ _____ = _____
　　　　result from step 7　　　result from step 9　　minimum calories per day
　　　　　　　　　　　　　　　　　　　　　　　　　　for healthy weight loss*

You now have an accurate, nutritionally sound figure to use as you start planning your menus, caloric intake, and weight loss program.

---

* If this number is less than 1,000, increase to at least 1,000 calories for healthy weight loss.

Appendix 3

Sample Exchange Lists

As discussed in Chapter 5, we at Structure House regard the American Diabetes Association's exchange lists as an excellent foundation for meal planning. (See pages 94 through 98 for a discussion of this topic.) What follows are sample ADA exchange lists that will give you an overview of portion sizes and the nutrition that they provide.

Note: The exchange lists are the basis of a meal planning system designed by a committee of the American Diabetes Association and the American Dietetic Association. Reproduction of the exchange lists in whole or part, without permission of the Americn Dietetic Association or the American Diabetes Association, Inc., is a violation of federal law. This material has been modified from *Exchange Lists for Meal Planning*, which is the basis of a meal planning system designed by a committee of the American Diabetes Association and the American Dietetic Association. While designed primarily for people with diabetes and others who must follow special diets, the exchange lists are based on principles of good nutrition that apply to everyone. Copyright © 2003 by the American Diabetes Association and the American Dietetic Associaton.

STARCHES AND BREADS

One serving provides approximately: 80 calories

15 grams of carbohydrate

3 grams of protein

1 gram of fat

Whole grains have approximately 2 grams of fiber per serving. Estimate a single serving size for foods that are not on the list, as follows:

Cereals/Beans/Grains/Pasta

Beans, cooked or canned, all kinds	½ cup
Beans, lima	⅔ cup
Cereal, cooked	½ cup
Cereal, dry, less than 100 calories per serving	See box
Couscous	⅓ cup
Pasta, cooked, all kinds	⅓ cup
Rice, cooked, all kinds	⅓ cup

Starchy Vegetables

Corn, cooked or canned	½ cup
Cornmeal, uncooked	2 tablespoons
Corn on the cob (6-inch piece)	1
Malanga, cooked	⅓ cup
Peas (green), cooked or canned	½ cup
Plantain, cooked	⅓
Potato, baked, boiled, or steamed	1 small (3 ounces)
Squash (winter, acorn, hubbard)	1 cup
Yam or sweet potato	½ cup

Breads

Bagel	1 ounce
Bread (whole wheat, rye, white)	1-ounce slice
Dinner roll, hard	1 small
Dumplings or gnocchi, steamed	2 small
English muffin	1 ounce
Pita pocket bread (6–8 inches across)	1 ounce

Saltines	6
Sandwich bun or roll	1 ounce
Tortilla (6-inch corn or 8-inch flour)	1

Combination

| Hummus (1 starch and 1 fat) | ⅓ cup |

FRUITS

One serving provides approximately:

60 calories
15 grams of carbohydrate
2 grams of fiber*

You can estimate the serving size for fruits that aren't on the list as follows:

| Fresh, canned, or frozen; no sugar | ½ cup |
| Dried fruit | ¼ cup |

Fruits

Apple, raw (2 inches across)	1
Applesauce, no sugar added	½ cup
Banana, medium	½ cup
Berries (blackberries, blueberries)	¾ cup
Berries (raspberries, boysenberries)	1 cup
Cantaloupe or honeydew melon	1 cup
Cherries, raw, large	12
Grapefruit, medium	½
Grapes, small	15
Mandarin oranges	¾ cup
Mango, small	½
Orange (2½ inches across)	1
Papaya	1 cup
Peach or pear (2¾ inches across)	1
Pineapple, fresh	¾ cup

* To get the most fiber from fruits, eat the edible skins.

Plums (2 inches across)	2
Raisins	2 tablespoons
Strawberries, whole	1¼ cup
Watermelon	1¼ cup

Fruit Juices

| Apple, orange, or grapefruit | ½ cup |
| Cranberry, grape, or prune | ⅓ cup |

MILK AND MILK PRODUCTS

Skim, ½%, or 1% milk

	8 ounces
One serving provides approximately:	90–110 calories
	12 grams of carbohydrates
	8 grams of protein
	1 gram of fat

Buttermilk, low-fat	8 ounces
Yogurt, nonfat	6 ounces
Soy milk (Silk brand)	8 ounces

Low-Fat

One serving provides approximately:	120–150 calories
	12 grams of carbohydrates
	8 grams of protein
	3+ grams of fat

| Milk, 2% | 8 ounces |
| Yogurt, low-fat | 6 ounces |

VEGETABLES

One serving provides approximately:	25 calories
	5 grams of carbohydrates
	2 grams of protein
	2–3 grams of fiber

A serving is ½ cup cooked vegetable, 1 cup raw, or ½ cup vegetable juice.

Beans (green, waxed, Italian, snap)   Okra
Bean sprouts   Pea pods or snow peas
Beets   Peppers
Broccoli   Sauerkraut
Cabbage   Spinach
Cactus leaves (nopales)   Squash (summer, crookneck, zucchini,
Carrots   calabazita)
Eggplant   Tomato
Greens   Tomato or vegetable juice
Jicama   Water chestnuts
Mushrooms

These vegetables have less than 20 calories per serving:

Celery   Peppers (hot, chili)
Cilantro   Radishes
Cucumber   Salad greens (all types)
Onions   Salsa (all kinds)

MEAT AND MEAT ALTERNATIVES

Approximately 4 ounces raw = 3 ounces cooked.

Very Lean

One serving provides approximately: 35 calories
                                             7 grams of protein
                                             0–1 gram of fat

Cheese (1 gram of fat or less per oz)	1 ounce
Chicken or turkey; white, no skin	1 ounce
Fish, fresh, frozen, or canned in water (cod, flounder, tuna)	1 ounce
Shellfish (clams, crab, shrimp)	1 ounce
Egg whites	2 whites
Low-fat/fat-free cottage cheese	¼ cup
Deli meat (less than 1 gram of fat per ounce)	1 ounce

Lean

One serving provides approximately: 55 calories

7 grams of protein

3 grams of fat

Cheese (1–3 grams of fat per ounce)   1 ounce
Lean beef (round, flank, sirloin)   1 ounce
Cottage cheese (4.5% fat)   ¼ cup
Salmon/catfish   1 ounce

Medium-Fat

One serving provides approximately: 75 calories

7 grams of protein

5 grams of fat

Beef, most cuts, trimmed   1 ounce
Cheese (5 grams of fat or less per ounce)   1 ounce
Chicken or turkey (dark meat, skin)   1 ounce
Pork (top loin, chop, cutlets)   1 ounce
Tofu   4 ounces or ½ cup

High-Fat

One serving provides approximately: 100 calories

7 grams of protein

8 grams of fat

Cheese, all, regular   1 ounce

Combination

3-ounce soy burger = ½ carbohydrate, 2 very lean meats
3-ounces vegetable and starch burger = 1 carbohydrate, 1 lean meat

FATS

One serving provides approximately: 45 calories

5 grams of fat

For heart health, choose mono- and polyunsaturated fats.

Monounsaturated

Avocado, 4 inches across	⅛
Oil (canola, olive, peanut)	1 teaspoon
Pesto sauce	2 teaspoons
Peanut butter	2 teaspoons

Polyunsaturated

Margarine, stick, tub, or squeeze	1 teaspoon
Mayonnaise, regular	1 teaspoon
Mayonnaise, reduced-fat	1 tablespoon
Oil (corn, safflower, soybean)	1 teaspoon

Saturated

Bacon	1 slice
Butter	1 teaspoon
Cream (half and half)	1 tablespoon
Sour cream	2 tablespoons
Sour cream, reduced-fat	3 tablespoons

Appendix 4

A Structure House Menu Sampler

Structure House provides tasty, nutritionally balanced meals to its program participants. The Structure House nutritionists and dieticians plan these meals in keeping with sound nutritional principles, and the chefs and their staff prepare a wide range of cuisines that are both consistent with these guidelines and delightful to the senses. Over the three decades of its existence, Structure House has hosted more than thirty thousand residents in its dining room.

To give you a taste (literally as well as figuratively!) of how good Structured Eating can be, here's a sampler of recipes from the Structure House kitchen.

Enjoy the delights and benefits of Structured Eating!

BALSAMIC DIJON CHICKEN

1 cup balsamic vinegar
½ cup Dijon mustard
¼ cup extra virgin olive oil
½ teaspoon black pepper
2 garlic cloves, crushed
30-ounce chicken breast

1. Preheat oven to 375°.
2. Combine vinegar, mustard, olive oil, black pepper, and garlic; stir well.
3. Add chicken and marinate for 1 to 2 hours.
4. Remove chicken from marinade. Place chicken in baking pan and pour marinade over chicken.
5. Bake for 30 minutes or until done.

YIELD: 6 SERVINGS

NUTRITION INFORMATION
Calories: 288
Protein: 33 g
Total Fat: 11 g
Saturated fat: 2 g
Carbohydrates: 7 g
Fiber: less than 1 g
Sodium: 582 mg

BROCCOLI MUSHROOM CHEDDAR QUICHE

CRUST
20 unsalted saltine crackers, finely crushed
5 teaspoons margarine, softened

FILLING
1 cup sliced mushrooms
⅓ cup broccoli florets, blanched
2½ ounces 2% cheddar cheese, shredded
4 eggs
½ cup skim milk
1¼ cups 1% cottage cheese
2 teaspoons cornstarch
1 teaspoon thyme

1. Preheat oven to 350°.
2. Make the crust: Crumble crackers and blend with softened margarine. Press mixture into the bottom and up the sides of a 9-inch pie pan.
3. Arrange mushrooms, blanched broccoli, and cheddar cheese evenly in the pie pan.
4. Combine eggs, skim milk, cottage cheese, cornstarch, and thyme in blender or food processor and mix until smooth.
5. Pour over the vegetable mixture.
6. Bake for 45 to 60 minutes or until internal temperature reaches 165°.
7. Remove quiche from oven. Let rest for 15 minutes, then cut into 4 equal portions.

YIELD: 4 SERVINGS

NUTRITION INFORMATION
Calories: 300
Protein: 24 g
Fat: 13.5 g
Carbohydrates: 21 g
Fiber: 2 g
Sodium: 560 mg

PECAN DIJON TILAPIA

Nonstick cooking spray
¼ cup light mayonnaise
¼ cup Dijon mustard
4 tilapia fillets, 6-ounces each
¼ cup pecans, chopped

1. Preheat oven to 375°. Spray baking sheet lightly with cooking spray.
2. Combine mayonnaise and mustard; stir well.

3. Lay fillets on baking sheet. Spread top of each fillet with 2 tablespoons of the mustard mixture.
4. Sprinkle 1 tablespoon chopped pecans over the coated side of each fillet.
5. Bake for 10 minutes or until fish flakes with a fork.

YIELD: 4 SERVINGS

NUTRITION INFORMATION
Calories: 270
Protein: 35 g
Fat: 13 g
Carbohydrates: 1 g
Fiber: 1 g
Sodium: 526 mg

PESTO TURKEY SALAD

½ cup light mayonnaise
⅓ cup plain, nonfat yogurt
⅓ cup classic pesto (see recipe below)
1½ tablespoons fresh lemon juice
½ teaspoon black pepper
16 ounces low-sodium turkey, chopped
1 cup diced celery
⅓ cup chopped walnuts

1. In a large bowl combine mayonnaise, yogurt, pesto, lemon juice, and pepper, stirring with a whisk.
2. Stir in the turkey, celery, and walnuts; mix well.

YIELD: 15 ⅓-CUP SERVINGS

NUTRITION INFORMATION
Calories: 90
Protein: 8 g

Fat: 6 g

Carbohydrates: 1 g

Fiber: 0 g

Sodium: 82 mg

Classic Pesto

2 tablespoons chopped pine nuts

2 garlic cloves, peeled

3 tablespoons extra virgin olive oil

4 cups basil leaves (about 4 ounces)

½ cup grated fresh Parmesan cheese

1. In a food processor mince the pine nuts and the garlic.
2. Add the oil; pulse 3 times.
3. Add basil leaves, Parmesan cheese, and salt; process until pureed, scraping sides of bowl as needed.

YIELD: ¾ CUP

NUTRITION INFORMATION

Calories: 60

Protein: 2 g

Fat: 5 g

Carbohydrates: 1 g

Fiber: 0.5 g

Sodium: 63 mg

POTATO CRUSTED SALMON

4 6-ounce salmon fillets

4 teaspoons honey mustard (or 2 teaspoons honey plus 2 teaspoons mustard)

8 tablespoons potato flakes, divided

4 teaspoons olive oil

1. Preheat oven to 375°.
2. Coat one side of each salmon fillet with 1 teaspoon honey mustard.
3. Sprinkle 2 tablespoons of potato flakes over the coated side of each salmon fillet.
4. On top of stove heat olive oil in pan over medium heat. Place salmon, coated side down, in oil and let cook for approximately 5 minutes.
5. Line baking pan with parchment paper. Place salmon in baking pan. Bake for 12 to 14 minutes or until the center just becomes flaky.

YIELD: 4 SERVINGS

NUTRITION INFORMATION
Calories: 318
Protein: 34 g
Fat: 19 g
Carbohydrates: 7 g
Fiber: 0.5 g
Sodium: 93 mg

ROASTED BUTTERNUT SQUASH SOUP

2 pounds butternut squash
¼ cup chopped white onion
¼ cup sliced carrots
¾ teaspoon garlic powder
⅛ teaspoon white pepper
6 cups water
1 bay leaf
6 teaspoons Knorr vegetable base (bouillon)
Parsley

1. Cut butternut squash in half and remove seeds. Peel squash. Cut squash into cubes.

2. Crush the bouillon cubes.
3. In a large soup pot add the squash, onions, carrots, garlic powder, pepper, water, bay leaf, and 6 teaspoons of boullion powder. Stir.
4. Bring to a boil and simmer for 1 hour, or until vegetables are
   soft.
5. Remove bay leaf and discard.
6. Puree soup in a blender. If any large chunks remain, strain soup
   back into the pot, then puree the chunks again.
7. Reheat soup to approximately 160°. Serve, garnished with
   parsley.

YIELD: 6 1-CUP SERVINGS

NUTRITION INFORMATION
Calories: 92
Protein: 2 g
Fat: 0 g
Carbohydrates: 22 g
Fiber: 6 g
Sodium: 653 mg

MELANIE'S SEASONED ROASTED VEGETABLES

Nonstick cooking spray
1 medium eggplant, sliced
2 medium zucchini (or 1 zucchini and 1 yellow squash), sliced
1 red bell pepper, sliced
1 green bell pepper, sliced
1 sweet onion (such as Vadalia), sliced
4 carrots, sliced
1 tomato, cut into wedges
1 cup sliced mushrooms
3 garlic cloves, minced
2 tablespoons fresh chopped basil

2 tablespoons fresh chopped cilantro
2 tablespoons fresh chopped parsley
¼ cup 2% shredded mozzarella cheese
¼ cup shredded Parmesan cheese

1. Preheat broiler.
2. Line a baking sheet with aluminum foil and spray foil with nonstick cooking spray.
3. Arrange vegetables on prepared baking sheet. Lightly spray vegetables with nonstick cooking spray.
4. Sprinkle garlic, basil, cilantro, and parsley over vegetables.
5. Broil for 10 minutes. Remove pan from oven, turn vegetables over, and sprinkle with cheeses. Broil for an additional 10 minutes or until cheeses melt.
6. Serve warm.

YIELD: 8 1-CUP SERVINGS

NUTRITION INFORMATION
Calories: 70
Protein: 4 g
Fat: 1.5 g
Carbohydrates: 12 g
Fiber: 4 g
Sodium: 75 mg

SPINACH CHEDDAR SQUARES

Nonstick cooking spray
1 tablespoon dry bread crumbs
¾ cup shredded reduced-fat cheddar cheese, divided
10-ounce package frozen chopped spinach, thawed and squeezed dry
¼ cup finely chopped sweet red bell pepper
1½ cups egg substitute

¾ cup fat-free milk

2 tablespoons grated Parmesan cheese

½ teaspoon dried minced onion

½ teaspoon garlic powder

¼ teaspoon black pepper

1. Preheat oven to 350°.
2. Spray an 8-inch-square baking dish with nonstick cooking spray.
3. Sprinkle bread crumbs evenly into coated pan. Top with ½ cup cheese, spinach, and the sweet red pepper.
4. In a small bowl, combine eggs, milk, grated Parmesan, onion, garlic powder and black pepper. Pour over the vegetables in the baking pan.
5. Bake, uncovered, 35 minutes. Sprinkle with remaining ¼ cup cheddar cheese. Bake 2 to 3 minutes longer or until a knife inserted near the center comes out clean.
6. Let stand for 15 minutes before cutting into 4 pieces.

YIELD: 4 SERVINGS

NUTRITION INFORMATION

Calories: 170

Protein: 21 g

Fat: 6 g

Carbohydrates: 8 g

Fiber: 2 g

Sodium: 434 mg

SPINACH LASAGNA ROLLS

Nonstick cooking spray

1½ pounds frozen spinach

2 tablespoons Parmesan cheese

1 cup part-skim ricotta cheese

⅛ teaspoon nutmeg

Pinch black pepper
½ teaspoon garlic powder
8 cooked lasagna noodles
1½ cups low-sodium tomato sauce

1. Preheat oven to 350°. Spray a shallow pan with cooking spray.
2. Thaw spinach and squeeze out excess juice until completely dry.
3. In a bowl, mix spinach with cheeses, nutmeg, black pepper, and garlic powder.
4. Spread ¼ cup of the spinach-cheese mixture along the length of each noodle.
5. Roll up and place seam side down in the prepared pan.
6. Pour tomato sauce over rolled-up noodles. Cover pan with aluminum foil.
7. Bake for 30 to 45 minutes until heated through.

YIELD: 4 SERVINGS

NUTRITION INFORMATION
Calories: 311
Protein: 19 g
Fat: 7 g
Carbohydrates: 47 g
Fiber: 7 g
Sodium: 356 mg

VEGGIE PITA PIZZA

Nonstick cooking spray
¾ cup red bell pepper, cut into strips
¾ cup green bell pepper, cut into strips
1 cup onion slices
¾ cup mushrooms, sliced
1 teaspoon dried oregano

½ teaspoon black pepper
½ teaspoon dried thyme
4 6-inch whole wheat pitas
1 cup low-sodium tomato sauce
4 ounces low-sodium mozzarella cheese, shredded
4 teaspoons grated Parmesan cheese

1. Preheat oven to 400°.
2. Spray a pan with cooking spray.
3. Add peppers, onions, mushrooms, and spices and cook until tender-crisp.
4. Spread each pita with ¼ cup of tomato sauce. Top each with ½ cup vegetables, and one quarter of each cheese.
5. Spray a baking sheet with cooking spray. Place each pita pizza on baking sheet.
6. Bake for 10 to 12 minutes, until cheese has melted.
7. To brown cheese, place baking sheet under broiler for about 1 minute.

YIELD: 4 SERVINGS

NUTRITION INFORMATION
Calories: 294
Protein: 17 g
Fat: 7 g
Carbohydrates: 45 g
Fiber: 7 g
Sodium: 558 mg

Notes

1. The Structure House Program

1. A. Bandura, "Self-efficacy," in *Encyclopedia of Human Behavior*, vol. 4, ed. V. S. Ramachandran, 71–81 (New York: Academic Press, 1994). Reprinted in *Encyclopedia of Mental Health*, ed. H. Friedman (San Diego, CA: Academic Press, 1998).
2. Centers for Disease Control, www.cdc.gov/nccdphp/dnpa/obesity/.
3. Jennifer R. Shapiro, Anna L. Stout, and Gerard J. Musante, "Structure-Size Me: Weight and Health Changes in a Four Week Residential Program," *Eating Behaviors* 7 (2006): 229–34. See also D. J. Goldstein, "Beneficial Health Effects of Modest Weight Loss," *International Journal of Obesity and Related Metabolic Disorders* 16 (1992): 397–415; Diabetes Prevention Program Research Group (William C. Knowler, Elizabeth Barrett-Connor, Sarah E. Fowler, et al.), "Reduction in the Incidence of Type 2 Diabetes with Lifestyle Intervention or Metformin," *New England Journal of Medicine* 346 (Feb. 7, 2002): 393–403; F. X. Pi-Sunyer, "A Review of the Long-Term Studies Evaluating the Efficacy of Weight Loss in Ameliorating Disorders Associated with Obesity," *Clinical Therapeutics* 18 (1996): 1006–35.

3. Get Ready for Structure

1. Adapted from the Weight Efficacy Life-Style Questionnaire (WEL), copyright © 1991 by the American Psychological Association. Adapted and used with permission.

5. Be Structured at Home

1. The American Diabetes Association's Web site, www.diabetes.org, contains a wealth of information about nutrition, including explanations of the diabetic exchange lists at www.diabetes.org/nutrition-and-recipes/nutrition/exchangelist.jsp. See also the Mayo Clinic's Web site for an excellent discussion of how the diabetic exchange lists work at www.mayoclinic.com/health/diabetes-diet/DA00077.

   Note: The exchange lists are the basis of a meal planning system designed by a committee of the American Diabetes Association and the American Dietetic Association. Reproduction of the exchange lists in whole or part, without permission of the American Dietetic Association or the American Diabetes Association, Inc. is a violation of federal law. This material has been modified from *Exchange Lists for Meal Planning*, which is the basis of a meal planning system designed by a committee of the American Diabetes Association and the American Dietetic Association. While designed primarily for people with diabetes and others who must follow special diets, the exchange lists are based on principles of good nutrition that apply to everyone. Copyright © 2003 by the American Diabetes Association and the American Dietetic Association.

2. The American Heart Association's Web site, www.americanheart.org/presenter.jhtml?identifier=851. The American Heart Association's Web site also contains abundant data, including recommendations, on a wide variety of nutrition issues; see www.americanheart.org/presenter.jhtml?identifier=1200010.

3. Nutrition information throughout this chapter derives from the U.S. Department of Agriculture, Agricultural Research Service, 2005. USDA Nutrient Database for Standard Reference, Release 18; see http://www.ars.usda.gov/services/docs.htm?docid=9673.

4. Siao Mei Shick, Rena R. Wing, Mary L. Klem, Maureen T. McGuire, James O. Hill, and Helen Seagle, "Persons Successful at Long-term Weight Loss and Maintenance Continue to Consume a Low-energy, Low-fat Diet," *Journal of the American Dietetic Association* 98 (April 1998): 408–13. See also James O. Hill, Holly Wyatt, Suzanne Phelan, and Rena Wing, "The National Weight Control Registry: Is It Useful in

Helping Deal with Our Obesity Epidemic?" *Journal of Nutrition Education and Behavior,* 37 (July 2005): 206–10.

5. Won O. Song, Ock Kyoung Chun, Saori Obayashi, Susan Cho, and Chin Eun Chung, "Is Consumption of Breakfast Associated with Body Mass Index in US Adults?" *Journal of the American Dietetic Association* 105 (Sept. 2005): 1373–82.

6. American Heart Association, 43rd Annual Conference on Cardiovascular Disease Epidemiology and Prevention, March 2003.

7. C. Marmonier, D. Chapelot, and J. Louis-Sylvestre, "Effects of Macronutrient Content and Energy Density of Snacks Consumed in a Satiety State on the Onset of the Next Meal," *Appetite* 34 (April 2000): 161–68.

6. Be Structured at the Supermarket

1. U.S. Department of Agriculture, www.cfsan.fda.gov/~dms/foodlab .html.

2. U.S. Department of Agriculture, www.cfsan.fda.gov/~dms/foodlab .html#see1.

3. U.S. Department of Agriculture, Agricultural Research Service, 2005. USDA Nutrient Database for Standard Reference, Release 18; see http://www.ars.usda.gov/services/docs.htm?docid=9673.

4. Margo A. Denke, M.D., Beverley Adams-Huet, M.S., Anh T. Nguyen, B.S., "Individual Cholesterol Variation in Response to a Margarine- or Butter-Based Diet: A Study in Families," *Journal of the American Medical Association* 284 (Dec. 6, 2000): 2740–47.

5. The Seventh Report of the Joint National Committee on Prevention, Detection, Evaluation, and Treatment of High Blood Pressure, www.nhlbi.nih.gov/guidelines/hypertension.

6. U.S. Department of Agriculture, Agricultural Research Service, 2005. USDA Nutrient Database for Standard Reference, Release 18. Based on cooked servings, visible fat trimmed. See http://www.ars.usda.gov/services/docs.htm?docid=9673.

7. Understand the Importance of Exercise

1. Centers for Disease Control, www.cdc.gov/nccdphp/dnpa/physical/measuring/target_heart_rate.htm.
2. Centers for Disease Control, www.cdc.gov/nccdphp/dnpa/physical/recommendations/index.htm.

8. Stay Structured Away from Home

1. The data quoted in this chapter derives from the nutrition information posted on the individual restaurants' own Web sites.

9. Maintain the Structured Mind-set

1. Siao Mei Shick, Rena R. Wing, Mary L. Klem, Maureen T. McGuire, James O. Hill, and Helen Seagle, "Persons Successful at Long-term Weight Loss and Maintenance Continue to Consume a Low-Energy, Low-Fat Diet," *Journal of the American Dietetic Association* 98 (April 1998): 408–13. See also James O. Hill, Holly Wyatt, Suzanne Phelan, and Rena Wing, "The National Weight Control Registry: Is It Useful in Helping Deal with Our Obesity Epidemic?" *Journal of Nutrition Education and Behavior,* 37 (July 2005): 206–10.
2. Robert H. Colvin and Susan B. Olson, "A Descriptive Analysis of Men and Women Who Have Lost Weight and Are Highly Successful at Maintaining the Loss," *Addictive Behaviors* 8 (1983): 287–95.
3. Herbert Benson, *The Relaxation Response* (New York: HarperTorch, 1975, 2000), 9–14; 169–82.
4. Edmund Jacobson, *Progressive Relaxation: A Physiological and Clinical Investigation of Muscular States and Their Significance in Psychology and Medical Practice,* 3rd rev. ed. (Chicago: University of Chicago Press, 1974), 12–24.
5. Jon Kabat-Zinn, *Wherever You Go, There You Are: Mindfulness Meditation in Everyday Life* (New York: Hyperion, 1994, 2005), 3–24; 70–90. See also Jon Kabat-Zinn, *Full Catastrophe Living: Using the Wisdom of*

Your Body and Mind to Face Stress, Pain, and Illness (New York: Delta, 1990); Sharon Salzberg and Joseph Goldstein, *Insight Meditation: A Step-by-Step Course on How to Meditate* (Boulder, CO: Sounds True, 2002).

10. Explore Lifestyle Change

1. Mihaly Csikszentmihalyi, *Flow: The Psychology of Optimal Experience* (New York: HarperPerennial, 1990), 2–12. See also Csikszentmihalyi, "Flow with the Soul: An Interview with Dr. Mihaly Csikszentmihalyi," *What Is Enlightenment?* 21 (Spring/Summer 2002), www.wie.org/j21/csiksz.asp?page=2.

2. Salvatore M. Maddi, "The Story of Hardiness: Twenty Years of Theorizing, Research, and Practice," *Consulting Psychology Journal: Practice and Research* 54 (Summer 2002): 173–85. See also Salvatore R. Maddi and Deborah M. Khoshaba, *Resilience at Work: How to Succeed No Matter What Life Throws at You* (New York: American Management Association, 2005).

3. Mihaly Csikszentmihalyi and Jeremy Hunter, "Happiness in Everyday Life: The Uses of Experience Sampling," *Journal of Happiness Studies* 4 (Spring 2003): 185–99.

4. Robert Ornstein and David Sobel, *Healthy Pleasures* (New York: Perseus Publishing, 1990).

5. Kennon M. Sheldon and Sonja Lyubomirsky, "Achieving Sustainable New Happiness: Prospects, Practices, and Prescriptions," in *Positive Psychology in Practice*, ed. P. Alex Linley and Stephen Joseph (Hoboken, NJ: Wiley, 2004), 127–36.

6. Adapted from Marsha M. Linehan, *Skills Training Manual for Treating Borderline Personality Disorder* (New York: The Guilford Press, 1993).

Appendix 1. Understanding Your Body Mass Index

1. Centers for Disease Control, www.cdc.gov/nccdphp/dnpa/bmi/adult
   _BMI/about_adult_BMI.htm.

Appendix 2. Understanding Metabolism

1. M. D. Mifflin, S. T. St. Jeor, L. A. Hill, B. J. Scott, S. A. Daugherty, and
   Y. O. Koh, "A New Predictive Equation for Resting Energy Expenditure in Healthy Individuals," *American Journal of Clinical Nutrition* 51
   (1990): 241–47.

Acknowledgments

Achievements are never accomplished alone. While I had a vision of what I wanted Structure House to be, that vision would not have come to fruition without the help and the education that I received along the way. This book reflects that vision. When I was first developing my interests in weight management and obesity, I was counseled not to work in the area. The time was the early 1970s, and the belief then was that obesity was an intractable problem. Professionals working in the area would not be considered serious. I was doing consultations in a hospital and was one of the few clinicians in my area willing to see people who were overweight. I was told that I shouldn't be interested in them because they were those "fat" people. As someone who had struggled with my own weight for many years, I didn't listen. On the contrary, I found the people I saw enjoyable and challenging. More important, I thought that I could be of help.

I want to thank all the individuals who have come to Structure House over the years and with whom I have worked. The number has now exceeded more than thirty thousand. With each one, I was able to learn a little more about this eating disorder. They have been my primary teachers. This book could never have been possible without them. Not only did I learn from them but they have also given me encouragement and sustenance in continuing my work. I cannot express the emotional rewards I have received by seeing so many do so well. In that sense, I dedicate this book to them.

I also want to thank my wonderful staff at Structure House, who have been so dedicated and so reflective of my vision throughout the years. Their tireless work and the concern that they have shown for our participants have helped to make Structure House what it has been and continues to be.

Nancy Freeman, R.N., BSN, C.D.E., our head nurse for more than twenty years (and affectionately called Nurse Nancy by our participants), along with Lillian Lien, M.D., provided the technical information to Chapter 2.

Marlene Lesson, M.S., R.D., our nutrition director, who also has been a part of Structure House for more than twenty years, provided countless hours of work, along with the assistance of Lauren Kruse, M.P.H., R.D., on the nutrition sections of this book.

Anna Stout, Ph.D., who directs our research efforts, focuses on bringing relevant research into the treatment program. Anna, while helping throughout the book, also worked with our exercise staff—Alicen Cisco, M.S.; Kim McNally, M.S.; Melanie Sweazey, M.A.; and Rebecca Grossfeld—all of whom assisted with the exercise material in this book.

Lee Kern, M.S.W., our clinical director, who has been with us for almost twenty-five years, has been tireless in helping direct our unique program and also contributed throughout the book. Lee, along with Trish Johnson, M.S.W.; Shula Lazarus, Ph.D.; and Deborah Klinger, M.A., L.M.F.T., provided information on the psychological and lifestyle sections of this book.

I also want to thank all the people at Fireside/Simon & Schuster who were always absolutely wonderful to work with and responsive to all my needs. Mark Gompertz, Trish Todd, Chris Lloreda, and Marcia Burch are a great team to have on your side. I particularly wish to thank the senior editor for this project, Nancy Hancock, along with Martha Schwartz, production editor, and Lynn Anderson, the copy editor, who all took this book to heart, doing such a superb job in reviewing and editing our manuscript. I could not ask for more enthusiasm and support in the writing of this book.

I also need to thank Mel Parker, my literary agent, who contacted me one day and said, "I always wanted to do a book about Structure House." How more flattering could anything be than to have an individual of Mel's knowledge and respect in the book publishing industry tell you this? His guidance and direction allowed this book to be.

A book of this kind must have a translator who can take the material and writings I have and translate them into the appropriate words for general readership. Thanks goes to Ed Myers, a wonderful wordsmith and author in his own right, who spent countless hours translating all our materials, dictations, recordings, and discussions with my staff and with me to make order out of it all.

Finally I want to thank four special people. First, Rita, my wife and partner for more than forty years, with whom I founded Structure House, has worked at every job at Structure House. Her heart and soul are very much a part of it. Second, I want to thank our three sons, David, Jason, and Michael, each of whom shared me with their younger sibling, Structure House, for so many years. As with all siblings, at a younger age, there can be jealousy but also love and concern. They each have developed into fine young men, each with a wonderful career, and they are still very much concerned about Structure House. I am delighted that they all continue to contribute to it.

Index

About the Author

Renowned clinical psychologist DR. GERARD J. MUSANTE founded Structure House in 1977 and understands firsthand the struggle faced by overweight people. After spending his overweight adolescent years trying countless diets that never worked, he devoted his professional life to developing and teaching the principles of behavior modification for overweight people.

Today, his internationally respected weight control program has helped more than thirty thousand people change their attitudes, perceptions, and lifestyles with diet, exercise, and education at Structure House, a residential weight loss center in Durham, N.C. Many celebrities, celebrity relatives, and notables in the field of business and government come to Structure House for its superior programs, integrity, and policy of absolute privacy.

Dr. Musante was the first person to adapt the principles of behavior modification to the eating habits of significantly overweight people and food abusers alike. Thousands of people have benefited from his methods and guidance at Structure House, where the behavioral etiology of food abuse is probed in a deep, uniquely successful way. Participants learn why they have been making negative food choices, and they move on to learn about taking personal responsibility for their food choices and habits to maintain a healthier lifestyle. Additionally, participants learn to identify and understand the antecedents of eating for nonnutritional reasons, developing personal resources and coping strategies to make successful changes at home. Structure House participants learn how to master relationships—with food, with society, and with themselves.

Dr. Musante's road to personal success—with his own weight loss and in his profession—began when he undertook the study of obesity as a psychologist at Duke University Medical Center. There he developed the techniques that not only enabled him to lose the weight but also keep it off. He says, "Once I realized that my relationship with food needed to change, and that food was for nutrition, not for comfort and support, I lost the weight and kept it off."

A respected leader in the field, Dr. Musante testified as an expert witness on obesity before the U.S. Senate Committee on the Judiciary. He also recently was chosen to serve on the N.C. Health and Wellness Trust Fund Commission's Study Committee for the Prevention and Treatment of Childhood Overweight/Obesity.

Dr. Musante received his professional training at New York University, the University of Tennessee, Duke University Medical Center, and Temple University Medical School. He is a member of a number of professional organizations, including the American Psychological Association and the Association for the Advancement of Behavior Therapy. He has served on the editorial board of *Addictive Behavior* and as a consultant to the National Board of Medical Examiners. He also continues to serve as a Consulting Professor in Psychology at Duke University and in Psychiatry and Behavioral Sciences at Duke University Medical Center.

Dr. Musante has authored many articles in professional journals as well as consumer magazines and newspapers. He has been quoted in publications such as the *New York Times* and the *Atlanta Journal-Constitution*, and has been featured in *Newsweek*, *People*, and *New Woman* magazines. Dr. Musante has appeared on national television shows, most recently including a feature segment on CNN's *Anderson Cooper 360*, and with Morley Safer on the acclaimed CBS news program *60 Minutes* as well as *Donahue* and *Good Morning America*. He also wrote the introduction to James Coco's book, *If I Can, You Can*.